High Performance
HEALTH & FITNESS HABITS
Engage Your Health and Fitness Auto-Pilot

MNOP Habits

M = Mindset
N = Nutrition
OP = get Out and Play

Scott F. Paradis

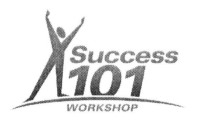

http://Success101Workshop.com

Books by Scott F. Paradis:

High Performance Health and Fitness Habits
Engage Your Health and Fitness Auto-Pilot

High Performance Habits
Making Success a Habit

How to Succeed at Anything
In 3 Simple Steps

Success 101 How Life Works
Know the Rules, Play to Win

Warriors Diplomats Heroes
Why America's Army Succeeds
Lessons for Business and Life

Promise and Potential
A Life of Wisdom, Courage, Strength, and Will

And coming soon:

Money
The New Science of Making It

Build Me a Son
A story of Hope, Love and Renewal

Be
A Messenger of Hope,
An Example of Faith and an Expression of Love

Are You Really Better Than Average?
Where You Stand and the Fastest Way to the Top

Change your life with these online courses and workshops
by
Scott F. Paradis:

High Performance Health and Fitness Habits
Engage Your Health and Fitness Auto-Pilot
www.Success101Health.com

High Performance Habits
Making Success a Habit
www.Success101Habits.com

Success 101 How to Succeed
Focus on Fundamentals
www.Success101Succeed.com

Money
The New Science of Making It
www.Success101Money.com

Success 101 How Life Works
Know the Rules, Play to Win

High Performance Leadership
Fundamental Leadership Habits

Loving 101
Making Love a Habit

Be
*A Messenger of Hope,
An Example of Faith and an Expression of Love*

High Performance Health and Fitness Habits
Engage Your Health and Fitness Auto-Pilot

Copyright © 2014 Scott F. Paradis
First Printing: December 2014
All rights reserved

The information presented herein represents the views of the author. These views may change. While every attempt has been made to verify the information in this book, the author does not assume any responsibility for errors, inaccuracies, or omissions.

Published and distributed by:

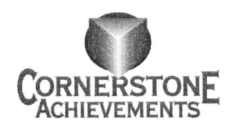

Cornerstone Achievements
New Hampshire and Virginia, USA
www.cornerstone-achievements.com

ISBN (eBook): 978-0-9863821-0-9
ISBN (paperback): 978-0-9863821-1-6

Published in the United States of America.

This book is dedicated to
every person seeking
to fulfill his or her potential.

This book is dedicated to you.

TABLE OF CONTENTS

Preface – 1

Foreword – 3

Chapter 1	**M**	You've Got the Power – 11
	N	Work the System – 20
	OP	A Complete Day – 26
Chapter 2	**M**	The Power of Habits – 34
	N	Stop the Madness – 43
	OP	Warm Up and Stretch – 50
Chapter 3	**M**	Believe then See – 57
	N	Why We Are Fat – 64
	OP	The Core, Bells & Balls – 71
Chapter 4	**M**	Attitude Determines Altitude – 77
	N	Fat Is NOT the Enemy – 84
	OP	Body-Weight Play – 92
Chapter 5	**M**	How To – 99
	N	Diet and Exercise – 106
	OP	Yoga and Pilates – 112
Chapter 6	**M**	Straw that Broke the Camel's Back – 117
	N	One Step at a Time – 123
	OP	Overcoming Resistance – 131
Chapter 7	**M**	You Are Not Alone – 138
	N	Take Aim – 145
	OP	Getting Up to Speed – 153

TABLE OF CONTENTS
(continued)

Chapter 8   **M** You Know What to Do – 162

                     N Eat Fresh – 170

                     OP Play Some More – 176

Afterword – 182

Appendix A: Health and Fitness Defined – 185

Appendix B: High Performance Habits Change Process – 187

Appendix C: Recommended Reading – 194

Appendix D: Feedback Request and Contact Information – 195

About the Author – 197

Acknowledgements – 198

About Success 101 Workshop – 199

HIGH PERFORMANCE HEALTH & FITNESS HABITS

Preface

Life is an opportunity; an opportunity to travel far, to travel fast, and to soar high. We can only make the most of this opportunity if we are healthy and fit. Aristotle once observed, "We are what we repeatedly do. Excellence then, is not an act, but a habit." We, you and I, are creatures of habit. Our habits make us who we are.

We naturally and most often thoughtlessly fall into habit patterns sabotaging our progress. *High Performance Health and Fitness Habits* is a program to change all that; to make health and fitness automatic. *High Performance Health and Fitness Habits* is not a motivational program. It is not a nutrition program. And it is not an exercise program. Though it focuses on mindset, nutrition and play, *High Performance Health and Fitness Habits* is fundamentally a habits change program. To fly high and fast and far your habits must be working for you not against you. To make a change; to re-create yourself change your habits.

Two Notes Regarding Style

First, by design you will find *High Performance Health and Fitness Habits* repetitious. Repetition is a tenet of learning. We build habits by repetition. I have attempted to walk a fine line emphasizing key points "just enough" to sink in, rather than "too much" to annoy. Please forgive me if I cross the line. Second, you probably have noticed my writing does not conform to AP style. My approach is informal, you might say conversational. Some sentences begin with *ands* and *buts* and end with prepositions. My intent is to communicate with you as effectively and directly as possible. Please forgive any lack of elegance. I hope you connect with the truths the words are meant to convey.

HIGH PERFORMANCE HEALTH & FITNESS HABITS

What if…

Do you ever wonder, what if? What if instead of procrastinating I embrace the opportunity? What if instead of rationalizing and making excuses I just move forward? And what if instead of judging and condemning and blaming, myself and others, I just accept what is and set about creating something better; a new me? Well, it's time to stop wondering what if. It's time to start making a change. Gain control of your habits and gain control of your life.

HIGH PERFORMANCE HEALTH & FITNESS HABITS

Foreword

The place to begin is always from where we are. Welcome to *High Performance Health and Fitness Habits*. Here we focus on developing and nurturing "MNOP" Mindset, Nutrition, and get Out and Play habits. In this program you will discover how to engage your auto-pilot to look and feel great automatically.

This *High Performance Health and Fitness Habits* program is divided into 24 segments organized into eight parts or chapters. Each part or chapter consists of three components; a mindset component, a nutrition component, and a play component.

We all want to make the most of ourselves and live full and fulfilling lives. Being healthy and fit allows us to make the most of the opportunity.

Health is the state or condition of optimum performance. We are healthy when all of our systems are functioning properly, as they should. When we are healthy we feel most capable and confident and sure, and we feel energetic and vitally alive.

Fitness on the other hand is a measure of conditioning relative to potential; or capacity. Everyone has great potential, but it takes conditioning to realize that potential. Conditioning is flexible; we can increase it when we need more and decrease when we need less. How much capacity we engage relative to our potential is a measure of fitness. We determine fitness by means of five elements: body composition, cardiovascular endurance, muscular strength, muscular endurance, and flexibility. We dial up or dial down the elements of fitness by means of the choices we make and the habits we adopt.

HIGH PERFORMANCE HEALTH & FITNESS HABITS

Start Down a New Path

You have made an important move, deciding to check this high performance habits program out. Now make a commitment to yourself to start down a new path, a path of high performance habits. Transform yourself and your life by changing a few habits.

I must ask you, right here, right at the beginning, before we begin in earnest, to consider something. We have been conditioned, and we often condition ourselves to approach learning as a mental activity; a function of intellect. Health and fitness, and by health and fitness I'm suggesting everything we cover in this high performance health and fitness program, has a total being focus. This program is not primarily an intellectual learning exercise. Developing high performance health and fitness habits requires intellect as well as emotional energy and physical effort.

Growth is a total being process. I'm asking you to consider right up front to go "all in". Commit one hundred percent to improving your health and fitness, your vitality and wellbeing.

By improving yourself, your health and fitness, your life will change. Not necessarily right from the beginning and all at once; but if you stick with it; if you continue down this new path; a path of health and vitality; changing habits will change your life automatically.

If you are a parent you know young ones are watching you, depending on you, and emulating you. Even if you aren't a parent; people are watching you, depending on you, and emulating you. You influence other people by being who you are and doing what you do. Help people. Help people feel better and look better. Help people get motivated to change by working on yourself. Not as a means of competition or a way to beat others, but to better yourself. As your health and fitness improve you will naturally be an example influencing others to take action. As you become healthier and more fit your body, your disposition and your activities will express what you can be; all that potential you possess.

Transform, refashion, and recreate yourself. You can.

If you have let yourself go, and most of us have at one point or another, you are going to have to overcome resistance; internal resistance to change. Your body has become used to taking it easy and used to dealing with the toxins you regularly expose it to. And your body has become used to paying the price poor nutrition and a sedentary lifestyle demand. Do the work of changing habits; those habits which have brought you this far. Start down a new path.

Jump in. Go all in. This is not an intellectual exercise. This is not about assembling and cataloging more information to add to your kit-bag for use later. Rather engage yourself fully and completely in building a better, a new you. Break bad habits and develop new, life enhancing habits. As you begin to remold yourself you will discover talents and abilities you have never tapped before. You have skills which you have, over the years, let atrophy. Put those skill and talents to good use.

There is no downside to this effort.

Well, I should rephrase that. By getting healthy and fit you become more capable. You can do more, give more, engage more and create more. But the process of improvement, the process of growth, of change, is not without discomfort; what some might call pain. You do have to pay a price. The new you however, will be well worth the investment.

Everything in life is constantly changing. And over our course in life we come up with strategies for dealing with change. One of those strategies is to cling to what we have and who we believe we are. The tighter we cling to what we have and who we are; which has brought us to this point in time, and our current condition; the more pain-filled is the process of change. The biggest hurdle to change we face is overcoming our own resistance. This can be a painful process. We cling to the way things are or we cling to the past and the way things were.

The greatest obstacle any of us face in changing habits; habits which may have, up till now produced only mediocre results; is ourselves. The process of change is an inside job. Your greatest struggle is always with yourself.

So start right here, right now, getting your head straight and focusing your mind. *High Performance Health and Fitness Habits* is a total being process. The change we are engaging in involves your intellect, your psyche, your social circle, and your body.

There is no stress-free, effort-free way around the minefield of change. There is however a shortcut through the middle. The way through is by means of a commitment. Commit to put forth the effort to change. To be healthy and fit, to be vibrant and full of life, to be enthusiastic, excited, engaging and engaged go all in; you must be "all in" for life.

Decide today. Decide for yourself. Decide to reach your potential. Decide now.

Express more passion and express more life. Do what is necessary to become healthy and fit; vibrant and fully alive.

Join with me on this journey of change. Engage through a series of small steps in a change process of immense potential.

Life is NOT a product of fate, luck or chance. Life is a process of overcoming resistance, of encountering hurdles; of engaging, of facing challenges; obstacles of all kinds. Life is a process of exploring and experiencing, growing and learning, and creating and contributing. You have nowhere to go but forward. You are headed somewhere. Why not take control of the journey, dictate the terms and go for the ride of your life?

Realize Your Potential, Get Healthy and Fit

To be the happiest you can be you have to be healthy. Being healthy means that your body is functioning properly and you are energetic and vitalized. Healthy doesn't mean you are the perfect specimen of power, grace and beauty. Being healthy means that on balance you have the right mindset, you fuel your body properly, and you overcome the natural resistance of life by getting out and playing regularly.

Some of us face extreme obstacles, treacherous challenges, that's just the way things are. We can't wish difficulties away. We have to deal with them, overcome them. While many people face challenges seemingly thrust upon them, most of us assemble the obstacles and challenges we confront ourselves. We set up our own obstacle course. Each impediment, each hurdle serves a purpose. The direction to go is forward; through the middle.

HIGH PERFORMANCE HEALTH & FITNESS HABITS

Don't look at obstacles and challenges as permanent impediments or as immovable roadblocks. Look at obstacles and challenges as opportunities to test yourself, as opportunities to change yourself, and as opportunities to grow. Grow bigger than the adversity you face. You have greatness within you. It's time to let that greatness shine.

It's not where we are that matters. What matters in this moment is where we intend to go and that we move forward; what direction we choose and what actions we take. It's not whether we are lean, strong, fit and powerful now. What matters is that we are moving in a direction to improve ourselves. We are becoming lean, strong, fit and powerful as we proceed.

You can be that person: someone who is healthy and fit, vibrant and fully alive.

We are in this together. Let's start from where we are and get moving forward.

We are what we repeatedly do.
Excellence then, is not an act, but a HABIT.
- Aristotle -

HIGH PERFORMANCE HEALTH & FITNESS HABITS

CHAPTER 1 MINDSET

You've Got the Power

What is the difference between the healthy and the fit, the active and the energized, the enthusiastic and the passionate and all the rest?

Do the healthy and fit have better genes? Were they just blessed with the right parents?

Were they raised in better environments?

Do the healthy and fit have access to things the unhealthy are barred from acquiring?

No.

Sure genetics contribute. Sure environment matters. Sure what we readily have access to, what surrounds us, affects our health and wellbeing. But the difference between being healthy and unhealthy, fit and unfit is something far more fundamental, something far more personal, and something far more powerful.

Think about this for a minute: How did you get where you are today, right now?

How did you get to the place, the physical location you are in this moment?

When you really think about it, if you are honest with yourself, you can see you got to where you are by means of a series of turns. Those turns, those changes in direction that led you to where you are right now, in this moment, were all decision points. You arrived at where you are right now, this instant, by means of a series of choices. You are where you are in space, this location, because of the choices you made.

CHAPTER 1 MINDSET: YOU'VE GOT THE POWER

Stepping back and looking at the big picture, that is, where you are at; your station in life; the same holds true. You got to where you are by means of the choices you made. You and I, we, all of us, arrived because we steered ourselves here.

Our health and fitness, our current condition in life is a sum total of the choices we have made up to this point.

This is a challenging concept, a difficult truth. You and I might not like to consider this idea, the idea that we each are responsible for getting ourselves here. We each are responsible for where we are, who we are and how we are. This concept, this truth is both potentially disheartening and magnificently empowering. But it is the truth.

The exciting implication of this idea is that if we arrived here because of the choices we made, that is we steered ourselves here, then where we go, what we do and who we become from this point on are a matter of choices we are yet to make. We can steer ourselves anywhere we want to go.

Look, we can't dismiss genetics or environment or the momentum of social influence. These factors impact our lives, the decisions we make and the course we take. This journey of life is after all a social journey. We are not taking this trip alone. We are intimately connected to the environment and to the people around us. Everything is connected and everything exerts some influence. There is a bigger story playing out and we are part of that grand epic. Life does happen and we are left, we are required, to deal with it. We are all swept along, to a degree, by forces beyond our control, but we are not helpless and hopeless. We are not adrift at sea; victims of prevailing currents and dominant

CHAPTER 1 MINDSET: YOU'VE GOT THE POWER

winds. We can navigate the currents and harness the winds. We are masters of our fate.

You have power. You have everything you need; everything you need not just to get by but to succeed spectacularly.

The first order of business when charting a new course is to accept full responsibility; full responsibility for the direction you choose, for the movement, the actions you take, and for the outcome, the results your choices manifest. Life is a choice and you make it. Life is a choice you make.

Now, this may not seem fair. Life may appear to be easier for some than for others. That may be true. There are valid reasons for those appearances. But none of that matters to you and me, to us here now. Our mission today is to change direction and become healthy and fit. So let's get to it.

Who Is Responsible?

You are meant to be healthy and fit. At times you might feel as if you got the one defective model off the lot; you were not issued a lemon. You came off the assembly line in perfect operating condition. Your body came with complete instructions, with pure potential for health and wellbeing. You have everything you need, built in, to be strong and fit, healthy and energized, passionate and vitally alive.

You have all you need. The question is: Are you willing to take charge and fulfill your potential? Are you willing to make the choices that lead you to health and wellbeing?

You have another decision to make.

CHAPTER 1 MINDSET: YOU'VE GOT THE POWER

I asked you earlier to go "all in" with this program. I asked you to commit yourself to a personal transformation; to remake yourself as someone who is healthy and fit.

Are you willing to take personal responsibility for this transformation?

To move forward, to become healthy and fit, determine the way ahead is up to you. Yes, you have been dealt a hand. Yes, you may be in a difficult position and have challenges to overcome. Yes, you may have to dig out of quite a hole. But you know, in your heart, no one can do this for you. You have to play your cards. You have to get out of your difficult position and overcome your challenges. And you have to dig yourself out of your hole.

You have taken a chance with life. It's time to start playing your cards; yes those cards in your hands. Do something with them. Move forward in a new direction. Embark on a grand adventure. A new day will dawn.

Where we have been and what we have done to get ourselves to our current state and condition are of no consequence. Only where we are headed matters now. Today is a new day, a new beginning. Put yourself on a new path by deciding, right here, right now, that your health and wellbeing, your fitness and vitality are up to you.

Okay, we have covered the most powerful and potentially far-reaching component of this or any change program: taking personal responsibility for change.

I AM RESPONSIBLE.

MY LIFE IS UP TO ME.

MY HEALTH AND WELLBEING ARE UP TO ME.

CHAPTER 1 MINDSET: YOU'VE GOT THE POWER

MY FITNESS IS UP TO ME.

This is a mindset, the mindset you must adopt to succeed in transforming yourself, in making yourself, in allowing yourself, to become and ultimately be healthy and fit.

High Performance Health and Fitness Habits is a simple program. It's a program about doing what comes naturally, about allowing what happens automatically. You have everything you need. You were preprogrammed for success. You have the potential to be healthy and fit. You have the potential to be enthusiastic and passionate and vitally alive. You just have to allow yourself to become and be. It's as simple as that.

High Performance Health and Fitness Habits employs MNOP habits as a means to reorient lives. MNOP habits are intended to guide you back to your natural state; that state of your full and greatest potential. Lots of things influence health and wellbeing: what we put in our bodies, our environment, the stress we subject our bodies to, the pathogens we are exposed to and so on. But nothing matters as much as the choices we make. And the choices we make depend on our mindset. The "M" of MNOP habits is MINDSET.

Except for a very small minority of people; those people dealt a difficult hand, there is only one reason most of us might be unhealthy or unfit. There is only one reason we might be overweight or flabby or weak and feeble. That reason is the choices we make.

Your Automatic Pilot

Life is a journey from point "A" to point "B". Each life journey has a beginning point and an ending point. Life

CHAPTER 1 MINDSET: YOU'VE GOT THE POWER

happens on the journey. Life is the journey. Consider this opportunity of your life as if you decided to take a road trip. Think of your body as your vehicle for making that journey.

Know this, you've got one fine vehicle at your command; a premiere model to use to navigate your course. You have control of a highly engineered, finely tuned, potentially high-performing means of transportation. This vehicle you now boast can do all kinds of things. It can move through multiple planes; twisting, turning, bending, contracting and extending. It can run and climb and jump. It can dive and swim and crawl. It can lift and carry and haul. Your body can function and operate in all types of environments. You can power your body with a wide variety of fuels. The human body, your body, is a marvelous instrument.

You possess this magnificent vehicle with awesome potential. Oh, and by the way, this vehicle of yours has a built-in auto-pilot. Yes, that's right! Your model comes with an automatic pilot. That auto-pilot is designed and intended to keep your vehicle flying high and straight and far. All you have to do is engage your auto-pilot and it will automatically take care of the details – it will keep all systems in tiptop operating condition, functioning smoothly; all systems go. Your auto-pilot attempts to keep you in balance, feeling right, and feeling as good as possible, given the guidance and support you provide.

Most people don't realize they have an auto-pilot so most never intentionally engage it. To be healthy and fit you can either worry about every minor detail of your journey or you can guide and support and let your body do what it does naturally. Make the right choices and let your auto-pilot take care of the details. Drive appropriately. Properly fuel and

CHAPTER 1 MINDSET: YOU'VE GOT THE POWER

tune and maintain your vehicle. Leverage the power of your auto-pilot.

When you make the right choices your auto-pilot functions as it should and your health and fitness are taken care of automatically. Health and fitness come down to choices people make.

Life is all about choices, and mindset drives our choices. So mindset matters most. Your primary task in *High Performance Health and Fitness Habits* is to develop positive habits of mind – a positive attitude and growth mindset.

You have the power to go where you want to go. You have the power to do what you want to do. You have the power to be what you want to be. That power resides in your mind. Use that power to ensure your success.

You make this journey employing, really relying on a marvelous vehicle, a vehicle with enormous potential. To realize your body's full potential make the right choices. First establish and maintain a mindset to optimize your body's potential. Provide your body, that vehicle, with the proper fuel. And tune, train and maintain your body to allow it to do all the marvelous things it is capable of.

MNOP habits are the most important components for achieving, sustaining and enjoying optimum health and fitness. Mindset drives choice. Nutrition is that process of fueling your body. And play is how you use your body; how you condition and train it.

Your body is your vehicle, your transportation. It is meant to move. Your body is a multi-faceted, high-performance vehicle designed overcome resistance and move through the environment. Your body will take you where

CHAPTER 1 MINDSET: YOU'VE GOT THE POWER

you want to go. It is meant to move, is designed to move and is intended to move, so move it. What you do with your body; how you move it, when you move it, what resistance you subject it to, what actions you take all matter.

Mindset, nutrition, and play are the three keys to health and fitness. MNOP habits are the essential elements of health and fitness; of performance.

High Performance Health and Fitness Habits is about tuning up your high performance vehicle so it takes you by the most direct route to a worthwhile destination. Engage your automatic pilot to ensure your health and fitness. To engage your auto-pilot we are going to leverage one other powerful tool, one other built-in process that guarantees results. That powerful tool is another advantage, another system everyone uses but most people do not understand or utilize effectively. That powerful tool is our habit process.

The Habits Process

We human beings are creatures of habit. Habits are our natural energy conservation mechanisms for achieving consistent results. If we choose, develop and employ the right habits; the right mindset habits, the right nutrition habits and the right play habits; our health and fitness are guaranteed.

This journey you are embarking on is an exciting opportunity. It's an opportunity to remake yourself and reorient your life. What we are undertaking, what we are attempting with *High Performance Health and Fitness Habits* is in fact simple. But this is the point to stress: you may not find the change process easy.

To change, to change direction, to get new results, new experiences; to become healthy and fit requires changing

CHAPTER 1 MINDSET: YOU'VE GOT THE POWER

habits. To change we must eliminate habits not serving us and we must develop and nurture habits to serve us. Changing habits changes lives. But changing habits takes effort. This means we will feel discomfort and possibly some pain.

In *High Performance Health and Fitness Habits* you have discovered the shortcut, the easiest and surest way to enduring health and fitness. But don't entertain any illusions. Adopting healthy habits is going to take work, painstaking work. Work you can do. Work you will enjoy, at least sometimes. This change is easily within your ability. You have the potential for greatness within you. You just have to want to change enough.

If you want it enough; if you want to be healthy and fit choose the right habits: mindset habits, nutrition habits and play habits. You can become healthy and fit. You just have to believe.

If you don't believe now, that's okay. Take baby steps. Start by taking action, doing something different. Change one or two simple habits. Once you start taking action and seeing new results you will begin to believe. And once you believe, anything is possible.

So, resolve, here and now, to endure the discomfort of changing habits. Do what it takes to engage your auto-pilot appropriately. Embrace the pain of overcoming your own resistance. Revel in the anxiety of overcoming your own fear. Make health and fitness a habit.

You've got the power. Put that power to use.

CHAPTER 1 NUTRITION

Work the System

Welcome to the first nutrition segment of *High Performance Health and Fitness Habits*. We are going to get into some specifics about food but don't be misled; this is not a cooking program. Our focus here is to change bad nutrition habits to good nutrition habits.

Nutrition, the process of fueling your body, driven by your state of mind and the choices you make, is the single biggest determinant of your overall health and vitality; your wellbeing. Deliberately abusing your body with poor eating habits leads to poor performance, lost opportunity, discomfort, disease and pain. We must get our eating, our nutrition habits right.

In these first few nutrition segments we focus on the big picture. Your mind, your mindset is your driver. Your mind is command central for the awesome systems operating your body. But your conscious mind does not have complete, nor even dominant control of your body's systems. Your mind and the choices you make impact and influence the functioning of all your bodily systems.

Our bodies however, are awesomely interconnected systems. The system we think stops at our skin is actually fully integrated with the environment and other multi-dimensional systems, some we consciously sense and many we do not. To help us understand the intricate functioning of the whole we often consider these distinct systems: the skeletal, muscular, cardiovascular, respiratory, nervous, digestive, immune, lymphatic, urinary, endocrine, reproductive, and the integumentary (skin) systems.

CHAPTER 1 NUTRITION: WORK THE SYSTEM

While all these systems are important and necessary components of who we are, in terms of health and fitness habits we are going to focus on those systems we exert the most conscious and direct voluntary control over.

Guide and Support

The body as an integrated whole has a command center, but understand the body is not a dictatorship. Life, living, even just in this multi-faceted, and extraordinarily complex and wonderful body, is a cooperative process. Many of our systems operate completely in the background, without need of conscious intervention.

The body is designed to function automatically. The challenge each owner-operator has is not screwing things up. To perform better, to be healthy and fit, to fulfill our potential we must collaborate with the automatic pilot optimizing the functioning of the systems of our body. We must develop habits to support what our body is meant to do naturally. If we can be a good collaborator; if we make the right choices and engage in the right actions; health and vitality are guaranteed, they are automatic.

As the driver, the operator, the commander of command central you can steer your body around all kinds of obstacles. By making smart choices and taking care of your body you fulfill your proper role: you guide and support. You do have the ability however, to drive the thing right off a cliff. Driving yourself off a cliff has immediate, dramatic and far-reaching effects. The fall may seem rather exhilarating and even exciting at first. Things may not appear to be all that bad for a time; wind in your hair, blood flowing, a great view; the effects of a bio-chemical high. The problem with driving off a cliff is the sudden violent stop at the end.

CHAPTER 1 NUTRITION: WORK THE SYSTEM

Most of us thankfully, avoid driving off a cliff. We don't do anything as obviously foolhardy or dramatically compelling. Unfortunately most people choose to take the slow road to decline. To keep this driving metaphor rolling… We forsake routine maintenance, and sometimes we deliberately steer ourselves too close to the edge. These kinds of behaviors, ignoring our body's best interests, failing to keep our systems in balance and failing to take care of ourselves, eventually catch up with us. Sooner or later we run out of gas or our breaks fail or our engine self-destructs.

We have each been given quite a charge. We have this magnificent, immensely capable body and this grand opportunity. Don't squander it. Take care of yourself. If you take care of your body; if you support it and provide for it, your body will take care of you automatically.

Your Body a Co-op

Human bodies are comprised of more non-human cells than human cells. Scientists cannot determine exactly how many cells make up a human body. Estimates range from the hundreds of billions to tens of trillions of what we would call human cells. But even our bodies are not distinct, separate, and self-contained. About 100 trillion microbes of all kinds call us home. Not that these non-human cells, these microbes, make up the bulk of the volume or mass of our bodies, but for sheer numbers we have more bacteria, virus, and fungi and other cells operating in all systems of our bodies than we have what would be, strictly speaking, labeled human cells.

Our bodies are one big cooperative. And that cooperative is tied into to larger systems along multiple dimensions.

CHAPTER 1 NUTRITION: WORK THE SYSTEM

Some, most of those microbes making homes in our bodies are good for us and some cause problems, especially when we allow things to get out of balance. This microbiome, as the scientists refer to it, need us to survive and thrive and we definitely need them.

We have our operating systems, circulatory, muscular and so forth, and we have this ecosystem which includes a plethora of others beings, microbes, all working in harmony to keep us healthy and fit. Looking from a broader perspective, when it comes to health and fitness, vitality and wellbeing, we must think bigger. We are actually tending a garden. We might just think of our bodies as being one big cooperative of systems and our conscious mind is potentially the most powerful contributing manager.

The magical thing, and it's a good thing too, is that the systems in the body, and the countless microbes calling us home, work automatically or mostly automatically to keep things functioning. The system is designed to take care of itself; given the right conditions.

Our bodies are truly amazing systems. They can operate in a variety of environments, from extreme heat to extreme cold. We can survive and thrive at various pressures but we definitely have an optimum range. Given the right inputs, the optimum inputs, the right environment and the right management our bodies and the systems of the body develop, regenerate, and function in near perfect harmony. We are meant to be well. We are meant to thrive and to be vitally alive. The cards are stacked in our favor.

If you'll bear with me for another metaphor. Our biological systems operate like programs running in the background on a computer. The system is pre-programmed to operate efficiently and effectively for optimum health.

CHAPTER 1 NUTRITION: WORK THE SYSTEM

The need however, is for at least adequate inputs and a cooperative, productive operator and manager; a driver who pays attention and makes the right choices; someone who effectively gages and manages the systems; someone who looks out for the best interests of the entire collection of organisms.

We, you and I, if we want to be healthy, heck if we want to survive, must listen to the systems. Become familiar with your own ecosystem. To enjoy optimum performance become a master farmer, a master motivator and a smart decision maker.

What you believe, what you choose, what you choose to consume and what you choose to do, impacts your systems, how your body functions. And habits are your main means of acting. Develop the right habits. Develop high performance health and fitness habits.

You Are the Driver

Your body is programmed for optimum performance, but it still takes its marching orders primarily from you. You are the driver.

Health and fitness begin in our minds but we haven't got far to go to arrive at our next most important contributor to health, wellness and wellbeing: What we put in our mouths. What you pick up with your hands and put in your mouth has a significant impact on how you feel and ultimately on what you do.

Nutrition, what you put into your body matters a great deal.

All of our systems contribute to sustaining and maintaining health, but certain systems have primary responsibility to ward off intruders and keep our systems in

CHAPTER 1 NUTRITION: WORK THE SYSTEM

balance. We call these our immune system, our lymphatic system and our integumentary or skin system. As powerful and important as these systems are nearly seventy percent (70%) of our immune function is found in our digestive tract.

What we voluntarily consume, what we ingest, through our mouths has a considerable impact on health and wellbeing.

Nutrition habits matter and they matter a great deal.

We've got a nearly flawless system; a system meant to carry us far. But we have to take care of that system. We have to manage that system. We have to support that system. We take care, manage and support our system by means of our nutrition habits.

Break the habits that hurt or inhibit your body's optimum functioning and adopt habits which allow your body to do what it is meant to do; perform at a high level.

Make no mistake. You were not issued a lemon. You are meant to be healthy and fit; vitally alive. Resolve to make smart choices; to develop the right habits so you can live healthy and be fit automatically.

Don't be the flaw in the system. Choose to fuel your body, choose to support your body, and choose to nurture your body with healthy nutrition habits. Once you develop those habits; proper nutrition habits; you can turn your attention to even more exciting opportunities.

You have the potential. The sky is the limit. It's up to you to make the right choices; to develop the right eating habits. Work the system. Guide and support your system with the right nutrition habits.

CHAPTER 1 GET OUT AND PLAY

A Complete Day

Welcome to the first OP health and fitness habits segment. The OP is short for **get OUT and PLAY**.

My mother, for one, doesn't particularly care to be outdoors. Not that she doesn't like the outdoors she just doesn't like the creepy crawly critters and flying pests we tend to encounter outside. And she doesn't enjoy the uncomfortable temperatures we sometimes endure living in the northeast. If you can identify with my mom, that is you prefer indoor activities, don't despair. MNOP health and fitness habits are not meant as a rule, rather the MNOP are intended as a guide to help you remember the most important components of health and fitness habits.

To achieve balance; to sustain health and fitness long-term, over a lifetime, deliberately build and maintain habits to nurture health and wellbeing automatically. This means a positive mindset. This means fueling our body with what it needs for optimum performance. And this means keeping ourselves; mind and body; actively, joyfully engaged in the adventure of life.

What I mean by OP health and fitness habits, what I mean by get out and play is to first break out of your old routines. Break bad habits; habits that don't serve you, habits that don't make you strong, resilient, vibrant and virile. This get out and play guideline is a tenet of health and fitness. Play is a way to free your self. Release your mind from everyday worries by engaging in joyful play. Vigorously engage in life every single day. Make play a habit.

CHAPTER 1 GET OUT & PLAY: A COMPLETE DAY

You know play has become a habit when, if you miss a play session one day, you just don't feel right. You don't feel at your best.

Every day is an opportunity. Every day is an opportunity to engage in the adventure. It's an opportunity to explore and experiment. It's an opportunity to learn and to grow. It's an opportunity to create and contribute. It's an opportunity to celebrate the journey. We do these best: engage in the adventure, explore and experience, learn and grow, create and contribute, when we are healthy and fit. Far too many people forfeit their health and wellbeing early in life to make a living, to climb the ladder, to secure a nest egg. These people give up health and vitality because they think they must to get ahead. The tragedy is after sacrificing their health, once they finally get ahead, once they believe they have accumulated enough to enjoy life, they then have to devote what resources they have amassed to trying to get healthy again.

Too many people trade their time, energy and talent; they trade their health and wellbeing for a promise in the distant future; a promise that for most never arrives. Don't sacrifice your health and wellbeing for an illusion. Take care of yourself now. Strengthen yourself now. Feel good now. The right habits make all the difference.

Train and Condition Your Body

The human body is designed to move; to explore, to express, to create. If you really wanted to be a couch potato, a spud, you would have been born one. If a potato is too active, then you would have been a rock, along for the ride. You aren't. You are here, an extraordinary being, in an extraordinary form, experiencing and expressing life.

CHAPTER 1 GET OUT & PLAY: A COMPLETE DAY

You have a wondrous mind and a truly magnificent body. Your body can do all kinds of things. It can take you places. It absorbs the energy of the environment around you. It can shape your mood, your feelings, even your destiny. You have the gift of life and a glorious tool, a vehicle, to help you navigate the journey. Put that tool to good use.

Oh, and one more thing; that tool, that vehicle, comes direct from the factory set for optimum performance. It automatically knows what it needs. Given the right inputs your body works diligently, unceasingly to achieve optimum balance and performance. You have an auto-pilot specifically set for high performance. Your task is to provide the right inputs to allow your auto-pilot to work its magic.

Given the right inputs, the right environment, and the right direction from a caring concerned driver the body will naturally and automatically respond. The body responds to demands placed upon it. The body develops and adapts to overcome obstacles, to keep up with the driver's requirements and to achieve phenomenal results. But the driver, you, must be actively engaged. You must make smart choices and you must provide the necessary direction and support. You are in charge. Don't take your hands off the wheel until your auto-pilot is fully and properly engaged.

Overcoming Resistance

If you don't ask your body to do anything; if you don't train it, condition it to move and to perform it will atrophy and whither. If you abuse your body, consuming toxins and poisons or punishing it with undue emotional stress and or physical abuse, you will age before your time. You will settle into an unhealthy weight. Your body will tire and break and you will invite all types of disease to consume

CHAPTER 1 GET OUT & PLAY: A COMPLETE DAY

you. Don't make that mistake. Take responsibility for your life; for your health and wellbeing.

Life, all of life, is a matter of overcoming resistance. This is a theme you are going to hear repeatedly throughout this program. We will address this more specifically again, but for now think of it this way: all of life is resistance training. This is an important point to realize right up front. Your body is a tool to overcome resistance. It responds to resistance. The more resistance it encounters; given the right inputs, which are fuel and encouragement and time; the stronger it becomes. You are your own personal coach, your own personal trainer. Training your body is your task. Train it well. Work together with the auto-pilot for optimum results.

Encountering resistance does create a feeling of discomfort, especially at first. Sometimes that discomfort may be extreme. We might describe the discomfort as pain. We can either determine to endure the discomfort and pain actively engaging in life or we can resign ourselves to enduring discomfort and pain as we age, wither away and die. The choice is a personal one. We make that choice by means of the habits we adopt.

Nurture a mindset a habit of embracing the discomfort; finding joy in the exertion; and reveling in the effort. If you can do this; joyfully engage; truly get out and play; then yours will be a happy life.

Get Out and Play

You may be wondering about this idea of play. Your body is a high-performance instrument. But for it, for your body, to be able to perform at a high level it must adapt to the stress of the load. All our systems work in an integrated fashion. You must push your body, and those systems which

CHAPTER 1 GET OUT & PLAY: A COMPLETE DAY

comprise it, to overcome the resistance of life: the resistance of gravity, the resistance of our mental inertia and our ever-present tendency to seek comfort and take it easy.

To get out and play consistently and deliberately, we must overcome our own resistance to exertion. This happens when we think, "Fun takes too much effort."

Make this thought a habit of mind:

It's not a complete day unless and until I get out and play.

Do something physically demanding, active, joyfully engaging every day. This can be as simple as walking vigorously for twenty minutes or more. Or in keeping with our theme of play it could be rough-housing or running around with the kids or grandkids for twenty-plus minutes. A good game of tag or wrestling or a water fight will do the trick. Rely on the kids to come up with something active; then jump in, get involved and stay involved.

Play might be engaging in any number of activities. You can run or jog, bike or swim, climb mountains or play games. By games here I mean sports. Games like basketball or tennis, ultimate Frisbee or racquetball, soccer or even touch football. Dance is a great physical activity. So, cut a rug. Get out there and groove. Or grace the ballroom floor.

As far as play goes, the point to emphasize is to exert yourself. Use your major muscle groups, get your heart rate up and engage your core. Get active, physically involved, for at least twenty minutes a day.

What doesn't count as play? What activities, though enjoyable and beneficial in other ways, aren't going to make the grade here for active play?

CHAPTER 1 GET OUT & PLAY: A COMPLETE DAY

Board games or cards, even if you play them outdoors; quiz games or social gatherings; and parties, unless you really do expend some significant energy dancing up a storm.

Bowling is a good activity to get you moving, but think about taxing multiple systems simultaneously for an extended period; not your liver from processing beer. If you are bowling with a group be cautious that you don't overconsume and offset the benefits of joyful play. Don't get me wrong; engaging, participating, actually doing something fun is of much more benefit than lying on the couch and downing a bag of chips, just be sure you actively engage. Move and you'll benefit from play.

Games like baseball and softball, though they can be very engaging, are typically played, at least in most recreational settings, for the social component. These are active events, but you may have to put a little more effort into them to reap the most rewards. Move around; keep active, stay involved in every play. Picking dandelions in the outfield isn't going to cut it. Do more to get your body into top form and condition. Do a little more to maintain an optimum level of fitness. So if you are engaging in games which might not work all your physiological systems, ratchet up your activity while you are out there. Be creative. Get moving.

Get out and play means engaging for at least twenty (20) minutes a day in an activity or combination of activities; what some typically call exercise. These activities tax your muscular and skeletal systems and work your cardiovascular and respiratory systems. By releasing your mind and engaging your body play energizes your full being.

CHAPTER 1 GET OUT & PLAY: A COMPLETE DAY

Play, real play, automatically causes your mind to relax. You release even genuine, legitimate worries. Your brain and endocrine system produce hormones which lighten your mood. Stress evaporates. Get out and play every day. You'll be better for it.

Mix It Up

Most people don't have the social schedule to engage in active games with other players every day. Families with young children are one exception. So for those days when you don't have a joyfully active social activity planned create an activity which provides similar benefits. This is what some, those not predisposed to engaging in play, frame as an expletive described by the words "exercise" or "working out". If you are one of those; someone who considers exercise an expletive; make changing this habit of mind a priority. Change your attitude regarding exercise by forcing yourself to get out and play every day. Once you make play a habit and begin to enjoy play's benefits you won't want to miss it. You just might not think of exercise as an expletive any longer; it's play.

To allow your body to achieve optimum health and fitness get active first. Develop a habit of mind to act. Get out and play. Do something, then over time begin to manage your play so as to optimize its benefits. You will get fit.

These OP health and fitness habits segments introduce specific types of activities or, here is that expletive again, exercises, for you to try during play sessions. Consider incorporating some or all of these activities into your play; your own fitness program.

You have a lifetime of health and fitness to preserve. Maintaining health and fitness is not a chore, an add-on or an afterthought. Maintaining health and fitness is an integral

CHAPTER 1 GET OUT & PLAY: A COMPLETE DAY

part of life. The specific play activities don't matter nearly as much as that you begin and continue to do something. Focus on and participate in a wide variety of activities at once, in an integrated, multi-dimensional program, or over time. To get the most benefit, emotional, psychological, physical and social make daily activities enjoyable and fun. Play every day.

Health and fitness depend on mindset, nutrition and play. Deliberately manage all three to stay healthy and fit. Guide and support your body to engage your auto-pilot. Establish and maintain the conditions, inside and out, for your body to do what it is meant to do and do what it does quite naturally: maintain optimum health and fitness. As part of this program, make it your task, your mission to play every day.

It's just not a complete day unless and until you get out and play.

CHAPTER 2 MINDSET

The Power of Habits

Do you have any bad habits?

Do you have a habit of procrastinating? You know putting things off, even important things?

I for one have been known to be a world-class procrastinator, world-class. I have put off all kinds of things and I have been known to put my rationalizer, my excuse tool, to extensive use. I can procrastinate and rationalize with the best of them.

Do you procrastinate habitually?

Right, jury's still out on that one.

Do you watch too much TV?

You may be thinking, "Is there such a thing as too much TV?"

Are your eating habits, shall we say, less than ideal?

Do you drink too much?

This is another one you may be thinking, "Is there really such as thing as drinking too much?" If you asked that question; you've answered that question.

Here's one: Do your exercise habits consist of crossing your workout off the calendar at the end of the day, as something came up, and scheduling it again for tomorrow?

Because, like my rationalization tool always says, "If I didn't do it today I'll surely get to it tomorrow."

Maybe we can answer that procrastination question after all.

CHAPTER 2 MINDSET: THE POWER OF HABITS

You may be thinking, "I avoid that problem of missing exercise sessions by never scheduling any."

Or you may be thinking: "How come we label these things: procrastinating, watching television, eating poorly, and skipping exercise, as bad habits when they feel so good?"

Let's be honest. We all have some bad habits. Bad habits are things we do automatically, without thinking, that don't serve us, don't move us forward. Bad habits set us back.

This can be an uncomfortable subject: bad habits. So let's take a new tack. How about good habits? Do you have any good habits, habits that serve you? To be more specific, do you have habits which advance your health and wellbeing, habits ensuring your fitness and vitality?

We all want to be healthy and fit and happy.

So, how come so few are?

The truth is most of us just put it off. We settle into comfortable routines. We develop and nurture habits steering us away from health and fitness. And most of us don't even know it.

We will get healthy and fit one day, some day. We are just waiting for conditions to be right.

Did I ask about a tendency to procrastinate?

Creatures of Habit

As we have already discussed, the vast majority of people are capable, and if the truth be told, predisposed to health and fitness.

CHAPTER 2 MINDSET: THE POWER OF HABITS

Anyone and everyone can feel and look better; can be healthy and fit and vitally alive. Health and fitness is, for the most part, for the vast majority of us, a choice.

We, you and I, are creatures of habit.

I have adopted and rely on habits, some good and some bad. Some habits help me stay fit and healthy and vitally alive. Some habits set me back. The choices I make; the habits I engage and empower; make all the difference.

What about you?

How is your health and fitness habit ratio: your ratio of good habits to bad?

Have you ever really thought about that?

Is your life dominated by bad habits: habits that disturb the functioning of your body's systems or habits that make you sick and weak and tired? Or is your life dominated by good habits: habits that strengthen and empower your body, mind and spirit?

We are creatures of habit. Roughly forty percent of our time, attention and energy are devoted to habits. These are things we do, processes we energize and execute without thinking.

Our habits have brought us to where we are now. Our habits have brought us this far. It is our lifestyle habits; our habitual mindset, our eating habits, and our play habits; which have brought us health and vitality or which have left us wanting.

If you are not as fit and healthy as you aspire to be you just might be giving more preference, more weight, and more energy to bad habits.

CHAPTER 2 MINDSET: THE POWER OF HABITS

What Is a Habit?

What exactly is a habit?

Let's take a second to think this through.

How do we normally approach life?

See if this makes sense, if this in fact corresponds with how you live your life, how you get through your days:

Life presents a circumstance; we find ourselves in a situation. Now, there is something common to all human beings, something we all, every one of us experiences. I use the word "feel" or "feeling" to describe this phenomenon. We confront a situation. It could be something mundane and simple or it could be something unusual and complex. Given a situation we feel a feeling, an urge, what we might call a desire or craving. That craving starts us down a path. We want to satisfy that craving so we define a goal. We begin to seek a reward.

For purposes of this illustration let's make this craving something simple and ordinary: we are hungry. We want to satisfy a hunger craving. We want to achieve a reward. We want to eliminate that hunger pang, feel full or satisfied or at least not hungry.

So a situation causes a feeling; a desire, a craving. When we have that feeling we usually thoughtfully consider options. We weigh pros and cons. In this case, we are hungry so we consider healthy choices. Are we watching our weight? Are we concerned about calories? Are we concerned about sugar or trans fats or other harmful food additives? Are we closing in on mealtime?

A situation caused a feeling which we can characterize as a desire. We thoughtfully consider options and then we

CHAPTER 2 MINDSET: THE POWER OF HABITS

act. We, of course, choose the healthful salad or nuts or all natural jerky to satisfy that hunger pang; to be our reward.

Isn't that how our decision process, our stimulus–response sequence works?

We have a situation, a circumstance. In this case we haven't eaten in a while and our blood sugar is low. We feel depleted, perhaps our stomach is growling. That circumstance has evoked a feeling; a hunger pang or craving. We thoughtfully reflect on available options so as to make an informed choice, the best choice, the right choice. After careful, thoughtful consideration we act, we have a meal, grab some food or devour a snack: we take action to satisfy our hunger.

Does this process make sense: we move from desire to thought to action to reward? Isn't that how our decision process works, typically, usually, mostly?

Hardly!

What really happens, most of the time is: we confront a situation; we feel a desire, a longing, a craving; an impetus for action. Then we automatically, thoughtlessly act.

We grab a bag of chips or some cookies or we venture into the freezer searching for ice cream.

Once we thoughtlessly satisfy that craving; once we've received our reward, we rationalize our action. The cookies were conveniently available. That processed, high-sugar snack fit the bill and saved us some time. Those cookies tasted great. You know what I'm talking about.

Health, weight, fitness and longevity, none of these factors came into the picture.

CHAPTER 2 MINDSET: THE POWER OF HABITS

We don't go from feeling (craving or desire), to thought, to action. We go from desire to action and only involve thought if we have to rationalize our choice after the fact. We do this in virtually every area of our lives.

Does that make sense?

We feel, we act. It's usually as simple as that.

This stimulus–response sequence driving our lives is our habit process at work.

Energy Conservation Device

Thinking is quite possibly the most difficult of all human endeavors. It is so difficult most of us will do anything and everything to avoid engaging in thought.

A recent study tested just how much people enjoy thinking. Human subjects were isolated in a room. They were asked to sit and think for brief stretches of time, just a few minutes. These test subjects were hooked up to electrodes. Their task was to think, but if they found that thinking was too challenging they had access to a button whereby instead of thinking they could shock themselves. Yes, give themselves electric shocks.

So the choice was: think or shock. How do you think this experiment turned out?

The test subjects could either think quietly, reflectively, deliberately or they could shock themselves.

Overwhelmingly the people chose to shock themselves.

We human beings just don't like to think. Thinking takes too much time, too much effort, and too much energy. Thinking is hard.

CHAPTER 2 MINDSET: THE POWER OF HABITS

We have a strategy to avoid thinking; to conserve energy. That strategy is called habits. We are creatures of habit. Habits are our built-in energy conservation device.

Don't get me wrong. Habits can be transformative agents. Habits can accelerate our progress; move us forward farther, faster, consistently and deliberately. That is how consistently high achievers get to be consistently high achievers. They put the right habits to work for their success. The right habits can be a ticket to health and fitness and to unparalleled achievement. Or habits can keep us stuck, wallowing in mediocrity; in illness, discomfort and disease.

Habits are a process whereby we eliminate thinking altogether from our stimulus–response sequence. We deliberately take thought out of the equation.

The Habit Cycle

We build habits one step at a time. We confront a situation, a circumstance. That situation generates a desire or craving. The first time we encounter this desire we have to look for and consider options. We might have to observe how others confront similar circumstances. We might have to actually think. After some thought, observation and deliberation we settle on a course of action and act. If we are successful we achieve our goal, we satisfy that craving. The next time we find ourselves in a similar situation and we feel that desire, that craving again, we recall the last successful process we engaged to receive satisfaction, to get that reward we seek, that feeling. We take the same action. We repeat the sequence.

Given a specific desire and similar conditions we initiate that same response sequence over and over again. If

CHAPTER 2 MINDSET: THE POWER OF HABITS

we get the coveted reward we incrementally remove thought from the equation all together.

We have a situation that causes a desire, a craving, and we have a pre-determined action path to follow to satisfy the urge. We have created a habit. Not thought required.

A desire leads straight to a predetermined action. We eliminate thought from the sequence and a habit is born. A habit is an action sequence we engage automatically, thoughtlessly, to satisfy a craving. We go from craving straight to action.

Habits are Automatic

We develop habits for all kinds of things, and this includes health and wellbeing. We have mindset habits influencing our moods and determining our choices, our actions. We have eating habits and play habits. These habits are routines moving us forward or setting us back.

Take inventory and you will discover habits are in many cases your prime movers.

Are your habits serving you or setting you back?

You can live deliberately, consciously approaching every moment of your life. You have the ability to think through every option and settle on the best moods, the best food choices and the most growth-oriented and healthy play activities every day. Or you can conserve some energy and make health and fitness a habit. Choose to develop and nurture habits to move your forward, habits to accelerate your progress, and habits to engage and empower your automatic pilot.

CHAPTER 2 MINDSET: THE POWER OF HABITS

Use your habits process not as an excuse for failure but as tool sustaining and ever improving your health and fitness.

Your life is already on automatic pilot. The habits you now rely on are taking you somewhere. Are you headed in the right direction?

Conduct a habits inventory.

Deliberately and intentionally replace habits that are not now serving you with high performance health and fitness habits.

Develop a positive attitude and a growth-oriented mindset. Develop healthy eating habits. Get out and play every day.

Health and fitness are a matter of habit. It's not a question of ability. It's not that some people are blessed and others are cursed.

You can be so much more; more capable, healthier and more fit. Choose to be. Make your habits serve you. Leverage the power of habits.

CHAPTER 2 NUTRITION

Stop the Madness

Sometimes we make health and fitness so complex; too complex. The more complex we make it, the more difficult it becomes in our minds, to sustain and maintain. We are often left to throw our hands up in the air, forget the "experts" advice and stumble forward or worse yet, settle for mediocrity. And in the United States that means pack on the pounds, reduce our mobility, trim back our lifespan, and endure an ever-growing string of aches and pains and chronic diseases.

If there is anything in health and fitness we love to make complex it is nutrition. We make nutrition so complex in fact that one has to be highly intelligent and extremely well informed just to be undecided and confused. Isn't that how you feel sometimes? I know that's how I feel; especially when constantly bombarded with conflicting opinions, conflicting research, and the diverse recommendation of competing interests.

Well, *High Performance Health and Fitness Habits* is a program to simplify.

High performance is not synonymous with complexity. We can do so much better by making a few simple adjustments. We can lose weight. We can become lean and fit and strong. We can put our body to good use to ultimately help us live a fuller, more fulfilling life. Success, prosperity and happiness begin with health.

Premium Fuel

Think of your body as a finely tuned machine, here's that automobile analogy again, like a racecar or to raise our

CHAPTER 2 NUTRITION: STOP THE MADNESS

sights and expand our horizons, a performance airplane. Our bodies are adaptable and flexible. A body can survive on quite a variety of inputs. To thrive however, we need the best inputs. Like a racecar or performance airplane our bodies perform best when operating on premium fuel.

You wouldn't put sand in the gas tank of a car or an airplane and hope to get very far. You could have a Lamborghini or a Ferrari or a top-of-the-line fighter jet. If you put sand in the fuel tank you will end up with an oversized paperweight. A finely tuned machine requires the right fuel and the right lubricants to operate at all. If we provide our vehicles with the optimum fuel, with premium fuel and lubricants, they perform even better. The same holds true for our bodies.

Nutrition is a matter of feeding our body what it needs to operate. High performance nutrition is a matter of providing our body what it needs to perform at its best. Nutrition here covers the gamut of everything we put into our bodies, this includes foods, beverages and other liquids, supplements, medicinal drugs, recreational drugs, and things we might inhale or suck on; everything we put into our bodies.

You might be thinking, "Here's the point in the program where we introduce that long list of things you should be eating." Not quite.

Stop Hurting Yourself

Progress is often not a matter of doing or adding more. Sometimes we make better progress by not doing certain things or stopping the things that are hindering or harming us. So we begin our focus on nutrition with the list of what to stop.

CHAPTER 2 NUTRITION: STOP THE MADNESS

If you smoke cigarettes or marijuana or anything else; if you use drugs of any kind, recreational, illegal or those not specifically prescribed to treat a condition; if you drink alcohol excessively, and by excessively I mean more than two drinks per day, stop it. Stop poisoning your body. You are destroying your life and the lives of those people around you. Stop it right now. Smoking or drinking is the first habit to break.

Quitting is easier said than done. On average it takes seven attempts to quit smoking cigarettes. We have all kinds of issues, emotional, social, and psychological tied up with our inclinations to abuse substances. But if you are serious about getting healthy and fit; if you are serious about being an example for those you love, STOP THE MADNESS.

As for alcohol, only a few alcoholic beverages are in any way beneficial, and these are only beneficial in moderation. The obvious one, the one extensive research points to as being of benefit is red wine. Different studies suggest certain types of red wine are better than others. The bottom line; if you enjoy alcoholic beverages make red wine your beverage of choice in moderation; not more than a couple of glasses a day. Sorry, you are not going to find much benefit in beer or hard liquor. To be fit and healthy over your lifetime take care of your body and break the drinking habit.

Get yourself some help and change those self-destructive habits: smoking, drinking, and using drugs, now.

Getting past the obvious toxins, the obvious poisons we consume, there are some other substances, foods and drinks, we need to stop using and abusing if we want to be healthy and fit. Remember, creating a new you is all about choosing

CHAPTER 2 NUTRITION: STOP THE MADNESS

and developing the right habits, the right habits of mind, the right nutrition habits and the right play habits.

We all have bad habits. Begin eliminating some bad nutrition habits.

Stop the soda. Don't try to rationalize that it's all about calories and diet sodas are the elixir of redemption. Those artificial sweeteners are throwing your body out of whack. Develop a soda reduction plan immediately and implement it. Break your soda addiction, your soda habit. Stop consuming soda and eliminate all related drink products; those with artificial sweeteners. If what you are drinking is made up of ingredients you can't pronounce stop drinking it now. Don't go down the road of rationalizing diet drinks. "How can these be bad? They don't have any calories." They may not have calories but they are wreaking havoc with your systems. Stop doing this to yourself. Get all soda out of your life.

Oh and by the way, don't plan on substituting fruit juices for soda. Fruit juices, even pure future juices with all natural ingredients, provide way too much sugar. If you are a fruit juice lover, cut back. Limit yourself to one small, no more than an eight ounce glass, per day.

So what does that leave? The most nutritionally sound options for beverages are pure water and green tea. You do, of course have other options, milk for instance, but the best options are pure water and green tea. You can, and I would recommend, smoothie's as a great liquid option assuming your smoothie is made with nutritious ingredients promoting health and wellbeing.

The painful and disruptive nutrition habit to break is a soda addiction if you have one. If you are drinking one or more sodas a day you have a harmful soda habit. Make that

CHAPTER 2 NUTRITION: STOP THE MADNESS

your number one bad nutritional habit to break. Figure out what might be triggering your soda cravings and begin implementing a new, more nutritious, habit routine.

Let It Go

Here is something to think about. We human beings are very averse to letting go. We will put out more energy and effort, we will fight harder, to hold onto something we already have, something we already possess, than we will to acquire something new. We know what we have. We are comfortable with what we have. We like what we have. It's ours. Change is a pain. But if you are not healthy and fit now, and if you want to be healthy and fit, then change you must. You must let go.

Stopping bad habits, breaking these addictions may prove to be the biggest hurdles you face in this entire high performance health and fitness habits program. This is not going to be easy, but it is doable. You can do. Make small changes. Adjust your habit routines. Two steps forward, one step back. Little by little start moving in the right direction. Work on your habits and eventually new high performance habits will make sustaining your health and fitness automatic.

Since I've been giving you nothing but good news in this section, here are two more categories of inputs to eliminate.

The first is anything with an artificial trans-fat as an ingredient. Typically these are hydrogenated or partially hydrogenated processed food additives. Trans-fats are inexpensive to produce and are used to enhance the taste, texture and shelf-life of processed foods. Manmade fats are killing us wholesale. After years, decades really of resistance many food manufacturers are recognizing the

CHAPTER 2 NUTRITION: STOP THE MADNESS

harmful effects of manmade fats to health and wellbeing. Manufacturers, some on their own, but many in response to pressure, are beginning to eliminate trans-fat ingredients from foods.

Look for trans-fat on the ingredients listing of the foodstuffs you have in your cupboards, pantry and refrigerator. Get rid of those items and stop buying and consuming foods made with trans-fat altogether.

And one final thing. I know, you're probably thinking, "Enough already."

I can assure you, you can eat a tasty, enjoyable selection of real foods; foods which will help you become and stay healthy and fit. But to make the biggest improvement, to start strong right out of the gate, eliminate what is harming you and your family first. Stop hurting yourself and life will automatically improve.

The final ingredient or category of foods or drinks to eliminate is anything containing high fructose corn syrup. High fructose corn syrup does not do you any good. Stop buying and ingesting anything with high fructose corn syrup in it immediately. There are other concentrated sweeteners out there. We shouldn't be consuming those either, but high fructose corn syrup is far and away the most prevalent and therefore most destructive artificial sweetener we consume. Let it go; get rid of it.

Well how to you like that. We have begun improving our nutrition by eliminating what is bad for us. It's all very simple, but not easy. Make a plan, a habits change plan, and little by little, step by step start adopting new nutrition habits. You absolutely will be better off for it.

CHAPTER 2 NUTRITION: STOP THE MADNESS

To support the optimum functioning of your body stop smoking, drinking and using drugs. Eliminate all soda and severely cut back on any type of artificially sweetened or even naturally sweet fruit juices. Eliminate any and everything with an artificial trans-fat ingredient. And eliminate any and everything containing high fructose corn syrup from your diet.

Our first stop: STOP THE MADNESS. You will be better for it. I guarantee it.

CHAPTER 2 GET OUT AND PLAY

Warm Up and Stretch

All right, if you haven't done it already, at least once today, it's time to get out and play. It's time to have some fun and move and groove. It's time to engage your mind, your body and your spirit in the dance of life. It's time to play.

Don't resist this idea. Make exercise, make activity, make play a habit. The key is: do something you love to do, something active and engaging, every day; something you genuinely look forward to; something that excites you.

If you have ever read Garfield, that cartoon strip about the lazy cat, you can probably picture Garfield responding to an opportunity to romp around with a sarcastic tone and a slothful grin. He usually responds to an invitation to move with, "I much prefer the couch." Being a couch potato, choosing inactivity over activity, choosing to be immobile over mobile, is choosing to be weak rather than strong, is choosing to be racked by aches and pains rather than being vibrant and energetic. These choices are habits.

We settle into a sedentary lifestyle because it is the easy choice. A body at rest tends to stay at rest. And, like Garfield, we rather come to enjoy our rest. If you want to be fit and healthy, if you really want to embrace this adventure of life learn to enjoy play.

Rest and recuperation, a nice nap, has its place. But keep this notion prevalent in your mind: Life is an adventure. You can choose to join in and participate. You can choose to engage and have some fun. Or you can choose to be a passive bystander. The world is not going to stand

CHAPTER 2 GET OUT & PLAY: WARM UP & STRETCH

still because you do. You have the ability to keep pace. You just have to train and condition your body to move.

If you make play a habit; if you get out and play every day you will be stronger, leaner and faster physically and sharper mentally. You will be more capable, more resilient, more intelligent and more focused. You are meant to play in this adventure called life.

Make this opportunity to get out and play such a powerful part of your daily routine that if you miss a play-date, a play session, if for some reason you fail to engage in some joyful activity one day, you will feel slighted. It's like you missed a wondrous event: a joyful family gathering, a fun-filled date or an exciting sports competition.

Getting and staying active over your lifetime is critical to the proper functioning of all the systems of your body. Play is a crucial component of your overall health and fitness, your sanity, your wellness and wellbeing.

Warm Up Gradually

Like before a great meal or an epic journey or an important exam, the place to start in every play session is at the beginning, with preparation. If you are not young and fit, and by young I mean less than twenty years of age, and by fit I mean already an athlete, you should never go from stop to full throttle instantly. Even fit young athletes shouldn't go from stopped to all-out effort without a proper transition and warmup. By jumping in you unnecessarily stress the systems of your body and risk injury.

At the beginning of any play session, of any activity session, of any exercise session, warm up and loosen up. Make an appropriate transition from inactive to active by managing your conversion gradually. Move from the cold

CHAPTER 2 GET OUT & PLAY: WARM UP & STRETCH

and tight state of relative inactivity into a warm and loose engaged state of play.

Begin by engaging your major muscle groups; those in your lower body and core. Walking or stepping, first slowly but then gradually increasing the pace, is a good place to start. Jog in place. Start getting the blood flowing and the heart pumping. Move around while gradually ramping-up your activity level.

Breathing is a key component of health and fitness. As you begin to warm up pull in fresh air. Breathe deeply, with your entire diaphragm. Synchronize your breathing with your body movements. Focus on inhaling fully as you relax your muscles and focus on exhaling as you exert yourself. Managing your breathing effectively helps you at work, at play and at rest. Don't forget to breathe.

Begin every play session with a few minutes of warming up; say five to ten minutes. Work those big muscle groups and your core. Get moving. Imagine yourself lengthening, imagine yourself centering, and imagine yourself engaging all the systems in your body. Pull more muscle groups in as you ratchet up your activity.

Jump around. Dance. Move, but don't flail. Stay controlled and deliberate. Breathe. Move faster and through longer ranges of motion to get your heart rate up. You are heading in the right direction if your breathing becomes more deliberate, more labored, and you begin to break a sweat.

A warmup is an essential, a critical component of every play session. Don't try ever to go from zero to game winning hero without inviting your body and all those systems, into the game. Make your warm-up a ritual. If a play session involves children, develop a routine with the

CHAPTER 2 GET OUT & PLAY: WARM UP & STRETCH

kids; a routine to rev-up the engine slowly over those five to ten minutes. Don't ever skip a warm-up. Stress, injury and or worse are what you risk by failing to warm up. No matter what the game, just do it.

The other necessary component of the pre-game, of the warm-up, is loosening up and stretching. You may have heard or read the research results showing that stretching before a run does not necessarily help conditioned athletes improve performance. Don't worry about those research reports. The thing to remember here is; you must invite everyone to the game. Engage all your bodily systems. Prepare for vigorous, joyful activity. Always warm up and stretch.

Relax, Lengthen and Breathe

After you have warmed up, after you've elevated your body temperature, increased your heart rate and begun to glisten with sweat you are ready to stretch those muscles. Once you are warm and loose you can play with abandon. Begin stretching gradually by engaging more and more muscle groups through continuously more taxing movements. Loosen and stretch out your muscle fibers and joints to get them ready to engage in the fun.

Increasing your range of motion during your warm up may be all the stretching you need for your play session. But to improve your overall fitness work deliberately on increasing your flexibility. This will pay a myriad of dividends including heading off injury and aches and pains in every aspect of your life. Stretch too during every play session as part of your cool down. Make stretching a deliberate component of your daily adventures in play.

Devote about five to ten minutes to your warm-up and loosing up. Devote about the same amount of time to

CHAPTER 2 GET OUT & PLAY: WARM UP & STRETCH

cooling down and stretching. If you want to focus on your overall flexibility allocate an additional five to ten minutes specifically to stretching.

You know what stretching is. You do it quite naturally. In your daily play session stretch deliberately.

People are naturally flexible in different ways. Some people can stretch their muscles and bend their joints through wide ranges of motion. Other people not so much. Don't compare your flexibility to anyone else. You can benefit by stretching and moving through a wider range of motion. So do it.

Here are a few things to keep in mind as you begin to focus on flexibility. Age, gender and body temperature all affect range of motion. You can't do anything about the first two; just know that the young are typically more flexible than the old. This is both a function of youth, the maturing of cells and systems, and a factor of lifestyle choices. We tend to move less as we age and our bodies adapt; we settle and our boundaries close in; we tighten up. And women are generally but not always, more flexible than men. As for body temperature; a cold body temperature is not conducive to stretching. Warm up properly before beginning to stretch.

Active and Passive Stretching

Experts in exercise science have defined a number of types or categories or methods of stretching out muscles and loosening up joints. These include active and passive stretching and so on. Here I'll bundle what some define with different labels and discuss three.

First is the type you are likely most familiar with, that is static stretching. Static stretching is a gentle, gradual lengthening of your muscles. When you stretch your

CHAPTER 2 GET OUT & PLAY: WARM UP & STRETCH

muscles statically aim to elongate your muscle for at least fifteen (15) or up to thirty (30) seconds. You can work through virtually your entire body and get yourself in all kinds of contortions using static stretches. Static stretches loosen up both muscle fibers and joints.

The second category of stretching is what is known as ballistic stretching. This is swinging or bouncing so that a muscle or joint moves beyond its normal range of motion. The motion of ballistic stretching requires the synchronizing of tension and release, of effort and relaxation. Because of this dynamic motion it can be a riskier technique. Be careful as you employ ballistic stretching techniques. You will become more comfortable with ballistic stretching over time, but begin slowly and gradually. You don't want to be pulling when you should be pushing, relaxing when you should be tightening, or extending when you should be contracting. We risk injury when we perform a technique poorly.

The third type of stretching has a fancy name, but you might just think of this method as a partner stretch. This method of stretching is known as Proprioceptive Neuromuscular Facilitation or PNF for short. This involves moving through the full range of motion in a ballistic way with a partner. The partner assists by forcing, force may be too strong a word, enabling slightly, ever so slightly, an increase in range of motion.

PNF stretches are normally a pulsing movement. If you are going to incorporate PNF stretches; pulsing stretches beyond your normal range of motion; partner up with someone who knows what they are doing and proceed with caution. PNF stretches can absolutely be fun and helpful for your flexibility and fitness. Just make sure you get the technique right.

CHAPTER 2 GET OUT & PLAY: WARM UP & STRETCH

Make a Habit of Easing In

Okay, we have focused on the first stage of every play session. Warm up and ease yourself into your vigorous, joy-filled, enjoyable and engaging play session. A proper warm up invites your entire body to participate in the party and significantly reduces the chance of injury during your play session.

As you warm up move your muscles and joints through their full range of motion and breathe. You can start at the top and work down to the bottom or you can start at the bottom and work up to the top. Just make sure you complete a thorough and comprehensive warm-up loosen-up session before you jump into your main activity. If you are not sure about how to stretch, or how to work on flexibility, look for a local gym or exercise class focusing on stretching and flexibility. Join in and learn to loosen up.

Though stretching, deliberately elongating your muscles at the beginning of a workout will not necessarily improve performance; definitely find a place for a deliberate stretching routine in your play sessions. Flexibility is an important component of overall fitness. Work on your flexibility consistently and deliberately. You will feel better, you will look better and ultimately you will perform better in every area of your life.

Be sure to warm up and stretch when you get out and play every day. Make a habit of it!

CHAPTER 3 MINDSET

Believe then See

See it and then you will believe it. Isn't that the way it typically works?

I will consider myself fit and healthy, lean and strong, skilled and agile, vibrant and vitally alive once I look that way, feel that way, perform that way, act that way.

I will believe I am fit and healthy only once I see it.

Too often we wait and watch and hope and pray that the right circumstances are going to come along and that the stars are going to align to make us how we wish to be. We wait and watch and hope and pray that our tendencies shift, our weaknesses disappear, and our habits magically change.

We watch and wait and hope and pray, and what happens? What changes is our weight. We grow older, we grow heavier and we move less. Instead of expanding our boundaries and our opportunities life closes in. As we watch and wait what we once aspired to; the greatness, the excitement and the achievements; becomes little more than making it through another day.

You want to be happy. You want to be healthy. You want to be fit.

It's time to stop wanting and just be.

What We Live By

What do you believe in?

Do you believe in destiny?

Do you believe in the system?

CHAPTER 3 MINDSET: BELIEVE THEN SEE

Do you believe in yourself?

In life after death?

In God?

We typically think of the word belief as an opinion; our or someone's conviction about something: a state, a condition or system of existence not immediately susceptible to rigorous proof.

While we claim to "believe" things, the proof of what we believe is evident by what manifests in our lives. Beliefs, what we really believe in, shape what we experience.

What we believe matters.

Think about what the word "belief"; where it came from and what it means.

Belief is a compound word with two parts: "be" means "by" and "lief" means "live." Taken together, the meaning of something we "believe in" is something we "live by". It's more than a theoretical concept, a notion; it is an actual framework in motion. Beliefs drive our actions.

What we believe is not a fantasy; it's not a dream, or a wish or even a hope. What we believe dictates how we live our lives; how we feel, how we think and how we act. What we do, the choices we make and the actions we take are in accordance with our beliefs. The outcomes in turn, the consequences of our choices, good and bad, our actions or inaction in many cases, determine what we experience.

More than that, we sift the circumstances we encounter, the triumphs we enjoy, and the tragedies we endure, through the filter of our beliefs. We interpret this life journey through our beliefs. By our beliefs we determine whether we

CHAPTER 3 MINDSET: BELIEVE THEN SEE

are succeeding or failing in life. We determine if it's all worth it.

At Your Core

You can be more than you think, more than you believe you are now: healthier, more fit, more powerful and more capable; more vibrant and vitally alive. You can engage life confident and strong. Health and fitness and vitality depend on what we believe. To make immense strides and irreversible progress with this habits process you may have to change your beliefs.

Changing yourself, changing your mindset, nutrition and play habits; changing your habits of feeling, thinking and acting in simple and profound ways will cause your beliefs to change. Manage this change process well and you will be a high-performer.

To perform at a high level and sustain that level of performance over a lifetime build a solid foundation. That foundation is your core beliefs.

Core beliefs are your most personal and most powerful beliefs about this world, yourself, and your place in this world. Your core beliefs color everything about you: everything you interpret as a feeling, every thought you choose to entertain or dismiss, and every choice you make for good or bad.

Core beliefs are your basic programming, your operating paradigm, your default approach to life. Core beliefs dictate whether you interpret the glass as half empty or half full; whether you have to be ready at a moment's notice to fight or flee; and whether you can actually tap into and release your true potential: that as yet not fully

CHAPTER 3 MINDSET: BELIEVE THEN SEE

uncovered set of talents and abilities you possess but have not really explored or exploited.

You have much to share with the world.

And you have much to gain from your journey.

Believe.

Core beliefs are crafted over the course of a lifetime. You might have come into this world ready for action, ready to take on challenges, ready to move forward and create and contribute to life, but you immediately faced resistance. The resistance of this environment may have been more powerful than you expected. And you were surrounded by other people who influenced you more than you know. Those other people contributed to the formation of your core beliefs as well.

No matter what happened then and who influenced you how, what matters today is that you understand core beliefs are driving your train. Your core beliefs are dictating your habits and your habits are determining your health and fitness and vitality. To change course, to unleash your potential, to become all you can be in this life; to be healthy, fit, vibrant and fully alive, you must empower core beliefs. You must free yourself.

It comes down to what you believe. Your health, your fitness, your vitality, even your wealth, your relationships, your success in life all are a matter of what you believe. Get your beliefs right.

Core beliefs are, in current digital age lingo, your operating system consisting of three parts. The first part is your fundamental belief about this world. Do you feel this world is a dangerous, threatening place or a safe and welcoming place?

CHAPTER 3 MINDSET: BELIEVE THEN SEE

The second part or component of your core beliefs is about your self. Do you feel you are connected and capable, able to engage and navigate and overcome?

And the final part or component of your core beliefs is about your purpose. Do you feel you have a reason for being? Is there a purpose for your life? Have you got a place in this world?

How You Really Feel Is What You Believe

Taken together, what you believe about this world, yourself and your place in this world, constitute your core beliefs.

So, again: What do you really believe?

We determine or identify our core beliefs by observing how we live, how we respond to circumstances and how we respond to others; how we feel and what we in fact do.

How does your life look? Do you like what you see?

Beliefs manifests in two key ways. First, beliefs manifest through feelings you feel in your body. Do you usually, mostly, always feel good or bad? And second, beliefs manifest through the circumstances of your environment and situation. You got to where you are by the choices you made.

Is it time to change?

It is time to change. Though we resist change, life requires, demands really, that we embrace change. Life is on the move, life is constant change. We are on a journey from where we are to where we are meant to be. To change course, begin changing your beliefs.

Deliberately work on your mindset; improve your nutrition and get out and play. As your body changes, and it

CHAPTER 3 MINDSET: BELIEVE THEN SEE

will change automatically if you persist, you will build new habits, new ways of feeling, thinking and acting.

It really is a matter of "believe it and see it" not "see it and then believe it."

Changing core beliefs is no simple matter. We build our core beliefs over a lifetime and we will take extreme measures to protect those beliefs; whether they are right or wrong; whether they are serving us or hurting us; they are ours. Change your core beliefs and build a high-performance foundation little by little by changing your habits. Once you change your habits the results you routinely get will change; you will feel different and over time your beliefs will change.

Begin changing beliefs by changing what you do: the actions you take. Fashion new routines, new habits. Those new habit routines will generate new results. Empowering new habits will fundamentally alter the course of your life.

Though at times we succumb to doubt and fear, or mistakenly take a path of least resistance, recognize progress in this reality entails struggle and involves risk. Breaking bad habits and building new high performance habits takes deliberate focus and effort; real work.

It is time to act. It is time to change beliefs, to be what you really are, to become whole, healthy, fit and vibrant. The ultimate purpose of life is to explore and experience, to learn and grow, to create and contribute: to express more life. What you really and truly believe about yourself, this world and your place in this world determine how much life you express.

Stop waiting to see. Embrace life. Take action. Change your habits. Your beliefs will change and your life

CHAPTER 3 MINDSET: BELIEVE THEN SEE

will change. The prospect of change and growth, with all the attendant trials and tribulations, can be uncomfortable and at times painful. The thing about the process of life though is you cannot get from the start to the end without going through the middle.

Become healthy and fit, vibrant and fully alive by believing you are. Believe you are now or you are becoming healthy and fit, vibrant and fully alive. Take action; simple steps. Build new habits. Those habits will alter your beliefs. The stronger your beliefs the more consistent your actions. It's a reinforcing cycle. Moving in the right direction; adopting the right habits will lead you to greater health and vitality.

Make a habit of telling yourself every day, at every opportunity, you are healthy and fit, vibrant and full of life. Post sticky notes and reminders all over the place: on your bathroom mirror, inside the refrigerator, at your office or in your workspace. And focus on changing the habits that will make that belief a reality.

You are healthy and fit, vibrant and full of life. Make this your mantra, your mindset habit, and life will change.

Believe in yourself. I believe in you!

CHAPTER 3 NUTRITION

Why We Are Fat

You have a lot to do in life. You have a multitude of options and a world of possibilities to pursue. Choices are virtually unlimited but time is not. Stop doing things that harm and hurt your body. Stop doing things that set you back. Break your bad habits and stop the madness.

Life is a bit of a balancing act. On the one hand we have all kinds of resources and assets available to us. We have gifts and talents and the love and support of friends and allies urging us forward. On the other hand we have free will, desire, and a nearly overwhelming selection of paths and opportunities from which to choose. Every choice we make comes with an opportunity cost. When we commit anything to one option we close the door on other options, another direction we could have chosen. Too often we choose immediate gratification and forfeit long-term benefits. Every choice we make is an opportunity to keep ourselves in balance.

No matter what we choose we only have one direction to go and that is forward. Every choice we make is an opportunity explored, a possibility expressed and every choice we make is an opportunity lost and countless possibilities passed by.

Don't worry about mistakes or poor choices you may have made. Life is always and forever renewing. Each day is a new opportunity, a new chance to express life, a new chance to move forward, a new chance to live your grandest dream. Only concern yourself with moving forward. Let go of the mistakes of the past. Let go of regrets and embrace a new life, a new you.

CHAPTER 3 NUTRITION: WHY WE ARE FAT

We're in an N section of *High Performance Health and Fitness Habits*. The N of MNOP Habits represents nutrition. To be fit and healthy, to engage and empower our automatic pilot for optimum performance we must fuel our bodies properly. We must develop and nurture the right, the best eating habits, the right and the best nutrition habits.

It's Up to Me and Beyond Me

Before we move on I must stress what may seem to you to be a contradictory or conflicting point. Give this some thought. I may not express the words adequately, so please devote some time and energy to exploring this point.

Life happens as a cooperative journey.

We are players with access to ultimate power, but we are still bit players in a very large and complex unfolding drama. We are masters of our fate. We write our own script. We direct our own journey. But it's not as simple as that.

We, you and I, each control how our journey unfolds. On the one hand we have absolute control; on the other hand we willingly submit and subject ourselves to rules and powers and events beyond our control in time and space.

The paradoxical idea I'm struggling to express is that we are of God, God is us, but we are not the entirety of God. We are an expression of the Divine; an awesome manifestation; but we are not the totality of God.

We, you and I, are in charge of our journeys. We choose the course and we are responsible for what we experience, what we enjoy or endure, but this adventure is a journey into the unknown. The process, the journey, is larger, grander, more complex, and sweeter than we can comprehend. Life, your life is under your control yet beyond your control.

CHAPTER 3 NUTRITION: WHY WE ARE FAT

You may reject this idea that you are in charge. After all you may say, "I don't have what I want to have. I haven't done what I want to do. I am not the person I aspire to be. If life is under my control, why haven't I arrived? If I'm in charge I surely would have done a better job getting somewhere."

It's just not as simple as it might seem. We chose to place ourselves in time and space within a larger context, for a higher purpose. We welcomed the opportunity. We immersed ourselves in the adventure. We are stars of our own drama but also we are contributing players in a larger unfolding epic.

The challenge to moving ahead in life is to accept the paradox: life happens and I am in charge.

To choose our course and set the pace, despite the obstacles and challenges we might encounter, we must assume full and total responsibility for ourselves and our lives. We can't blame something or someone else for what happens, what we've experienced, what we've done or failed to do, or for what we've become. All circumstances, all events, all happenings, all people serve a purpose; a good and noble purpose.

Even if it doesn't feel like it at the time, life is happening to serve our best interests. If we are willing to embrace life, if we are willing to do what it takes and take hold of the steering wheel and drive, we well have a totally different experience of life than if we decide to live as a victim, a passenger.

Do you get the idea?

Do you see the challenge?

CHAPTER 3 NUTRITION: WHY WE ARE FAT

By recognizing we are responsible for getting to here; for our condition and our experiences up till now; we risk weighing ourselves down with judgment, blame and regret. Don't fall into that trap.

Life is not a punishment, life is an opportunity. Avail yourself of the opportunity. Create your adventure. Take full and total responsibility for your self; not for anyone else; and not for everything that happens. Take responsibility for how you feel, what you think about and what you do.

Taking responsibility is liberating. Free yourself to make wise, life-enhancing decisions.

The Choices We Make

With this paradox in mind: *We are totally responsible but not to blame;* know there is only one reason we are not fit and healthy. There is only one reason we are not living up to our full potential. That reason is the choices we make.

We have chosen the path. We have made our way to here. We are who we are. We've done what we've done. It's okay. We've done the best we could with what we've had. Now it's time to chart a new course.

Okay, we may be overweight; we may be weak and unsteady and unsure, but as surely as we've made ourselves into the person we are, we can fashion a new future. We can change our course, change our path and change ourselves.

Let's talk about the elephant in the room: Most Americans are overweight. Let's go there.

We are who we are because of the choices we have made. If we make new choices we will move in a new direction and generate new results.

CHAPTER 3 NUTRITION: WHY WE ARE FAT

Beyond the choices we make, the consequences of those choices are results. Overweight people make choices which invoke or empower one of three, or a combination of three primary contributing factors to pack on excess pounds.

The first, most common contributor and the factor cited as "conventional wisdom" by the health, fitness and nutrition industries and the factor believed to be the most prevalent cause of weight gain and obesity in America is a chronic calorie imbalance. That is people gain weight because they consume more calories than they expend. We eat too much, too much energy (a calorie is an energy unit), too many calories relative to our physical activity.

This calorie mismatch, eating too much, is believed to be the most common cause of weight gain. Excess calories are believed to be the cause of obesity, heart disease, diabetes and the legion of other acute and chronic health maladies now plaguing the United States and much of the developed world. In simple terms we, as a society, have gotten so good at feeding people, we eat too much. Alleviating hunger we are killing ourselves in other ways.

In America and in most of the developed world food is conveniently available in large quantities at relatively low cost. Food offers and provides a multitude of benefits far beyond nurturing and fueling bodies. Food gives us pleasure; life is what happens in between meals. Food pleases our senses of taste, touch and smell. Eating good food is an enjoyable experience. Eating food is a social bonding ritual. We break bread together to connect with other people. Food provides emotional comfort. Eating, when food is cheap and conveniently available, is simple and easy.

CHAPTER 3 NUTRITION: WHY WE ARE FAT

In an environment rich with food, we can easily out-eat exercise. It's easier to consume calories, too many calories, than it is to burn them off through physical activity, exercise or play.

This idea, that calories are the primary cause of obesity and the negative health consequences of being overweight, is a myth. Sure, many people eat too much; and many people consume for the wrong reasons. But calories, energy units of food, are not **why** we are fat.

Most people buy into the calorie myth. They count calories. They attempt to restore health and fitness by balancing calories consumed with calories burned through physical activity; through diet and exercise. Dieters attempt to reduce fat and trim back calories. People looking to lose weight spend endless hours at the gym, working, working and working.

Diet and exercise, like most people think of diet and exercise, gets results but over the long term just does not work. With diet and exercise we get short-term results but unless and until we change our habits any progress is fleeting.

Too often even when dieting and sticking to an exercise regimen people consume the wrong things. In the long run they just get heavier. Dieters exercise consistently and strenuously to get the upper hand temporarily. They see a glimmer of hope. But unfortunately because of bad habits they usually ultimately fail. It's not how many calories we eat that are making us fat. **It's what we are eating that is making us fat.** We are making the wrong choices.

The second reason and really the primary reason so many people are overweight is that their body chemistry is out of whack. Their systems are malfunctioning. Their

CHAPTER 3 NUTRITION: WHY WE ARE FAT

hormones have gone a-rye. Their bodies are overwhelmed by foodstuffs and inputs that have muddled up their systems. A mix of toxic inputs push their bodies out of balance. Smoking, drinking, doing drugs, eating the wrong foods, and succumbing to the adverse effects of stress damage the controls. Bad nutrition habits and bad lifestyle choices punish the body. We pay the price for temporary pleasures; pleasures which have become habits; over the course of a lifetime.

The third cause for gaining weight is similar to the last in that we throw our systems out of whack by eating the wrong foodstuffs and putting toxins in our bodies. Rather than throwing our hormones out of whack however, we mistakenly kill off components of that collaborative community we must nurture and sustain to enjoy health and fitness. Our bodies are built around our guts. Upwards of seventy percent of our immune system originates from and operates in our digestive tract. Poor nutrition instead of nurturing the community of good bacteria and other organisms helping us live and thrive kills them off. Upsetting the balance of healthy organisms in our digestive tract we throw our entire system into disarray.

When we do not habitually do the right thing, the best thing for health and fitness, we sabotage the functioning of our own systems; our own bodies. We destroy our health.

We are fat because we have made poor choices.

We have nurtured and sustained habits that hurt rather than help. But we are not destined to stay where we are. Change what you eat, what you habitually consume, and change who you become.

CHAPTER 3 GET OUT AND PLAY

The Core, Bells and Balls

We have stressed the point: health and fitness is a total being effort, a total being condition. Besides managing or supporting the systems of the body, our physiology, we must be mindful of our psychology. We also have to be aware that the social environment we put or find ourselves in impacts our health and wellbeing.

We have much to consider; much to manage when it comes to developing and maintaining high performance health and fitness habits. But remember, it's really a matter of stripping away the distractions, the toxins and the stressors, and letting our bodies do what they do naturally, automatically.

My intention with this program is not to introduce complexity into your life. We are after simplicity. It's not a matter of stressing over every minor detail; rather it's a matter of taking care of the little things which ultimately drive the big things. When we get the little things right the big things quite naturally take care of themselves.

One of those little things to build and sustain health and fitness is play. Get out and play every day. This is a truism: "Use it or lose it." Your body is meant to move. It's prepared to move. It's designed to grow and adapt. It's designed to withstand and overcome resistance, the stresses of this world. But if you don't put it to task; if you don't deliberately condition and train your body; your body is not going to be ready when you need it. It won't even be ready for the simple things.

We have established: We must move every day. We have highlighted the processes, the importance of warming

CHAPTER 3 GET OUT & PLAY: THE CORE, BELLS & BALLS

up and cooling down. Deliberately and consistently stretching sustains your ability to move through a wide range of motion. Now let's consider the core of strength, endurance, and flexibility; what holds it, you, all together.

It's All About the Core

You have hands and feet and arms and legs and a head. They all attach to your torso, your core. Your core is that area of your body from your chest through your abdomen to your pelvis. In addition to housing vital organs and systems, your core contains the skeletal structure, muscles and joints that allow your magnificent body to operate across multiple planes of motion; to twist, to turn, to bend, to extend. Your core both stabilizes and allows your body to move.

Muscles, bones and joints of your core stabilize your spine, maintain your posture and ensure overall balance and stability. Your core allows you to move fluidly and deliberately. Your core is the base from which your appendages, arms and legs and head operate. High performance health and fitness starts with a strong, flexible and fluidly dynamic core.

Before you lie down and start knocking out crunches, consider what movements we make which do not engage our core. Only small, slight movements like writing, or texting or signing with your hands or perhaps using your feet in an isolated way or making expressions on your face, do not rely on your core. Usually, mostly, almost all the time, even if the motion is minor your core is holding or stabilizing your body, that arm or leg, hand or foot or your head. Mostly everything you do, from sitting up, to standing and walking and running, to picking things up, and hugging your loved ones all involve your core.

CHAPTER 3 GET OUT & PLAY: THE CORE, BELLS & BALLS

Strengthening and developing your core is not necessarily all about crunches or sit ups. There are other more effective ways to work your core. Isolating the muscles of your core and working on them in a deliberate, targeted way is absolutely helpful. But, let's think bigger than that.

Virtually every movement you make; including engaging, joyful play; incorporates your core. Work your core as you work your entire body.

Tools to Consider

Where to start?

We will get to bodyweight and weight bearing exercises in later sessions. For now let's look at three tools and or techniques to consider incorporating in your daily play routine. These are not things you must do every day. It's just that variety is the spice of life, so spice it up. Look for play routines you enjoy. Incorporating these tools will expand your fitness repertoire.

The first item is the kettlebell. The kettlebell was developed in Russia in the 1700's. It was originally used on the farm to weigh crops; however, it was soon adopted as an exercise tool. The significant advantage of kettlebell training is that a kettlebell routine works virtually the entire body through a series of ballistic moves. Effective kettlebell training works your cardiovascular system, and improves muscular strength, muscular endurance and flexibility.

A well-executed kettlebell routine is a complete body workout and can be taxing. If you are just beginning to get yourself in shape, determine to get to kettlebell training after you improve your overall core fitness.

CHAPTER 3 GET OUT & PLAY: THE CORE, BELLS & BALLS

The kettlebell itself differs from a traditional dumbbell in that the center of mass is extended beyond the hand. The unique shape of the kettlebell facilitates swinging, ballistic movements. The kettlebell provides an unstable force for handling which taxes the body in ways unlike traditional weight lifting.

Kettlebell exercises improve strength and endurance and incorporate your core. Kettlebells themselves come in all sizes and are made from a variety of materials. Traditional kettlebells are metal, but you can get some now made of cloth and stuffed like a bean bag. You can even make kettlebell-like devices yourself.

Look for programs and routines to kick-off your kettlebell training slowly. Because of the dynamic focus of kettlebell training on your core, if you stick with kettlebell training your overall fitness level will improve dramatically. Give the kettlebell a try.

A Weighted Ball

The second tool or technique, or the potentially new component to add to your play routine is the medicine ball. Balls have been a staple of play for generations. We use balls of all sizes and shapes to engage in all kinds of fun. The medicine ball is just a weighted ball to incorporate in your play sessions.

The medicine ball, as an exercise tool, has been around for thousands of years. We can trace the use of the medicine ball back to ancient Greece and Persia. Medicine balls are still around today because they are fun and effective tools to improve overall fitness.

Like all exercises, proper form is essential for avoiding injury and maximizing your efforts. By stressing, pushing

CHAPTER 3 GET OUT & PLAY: THE CORE, BELLS & BALLS

your muscles and your body systems just a little bit, progressively, you signal your body to adapt and improve. Medicine ball exercises are another means to push yourself, to stress your systems.

You can perform a wide variety of exercises with a medicine ball alone or with other people. Incorporate medicine ball movements involving as much of your body as possible; the more muscle groups, from head to toe, the better. Engaging more muscle groups decisively employs your core.

Hold, toss or manipulate the medicine ball as you move through multiple planes of motion in a dynamic way. By moving through multiple planes of motion you just cannot leave your core out. The more you tax your core, more intensely and with proper form and technique, the better off you will be. Try using some medicine balls in your daily play sessions.

Deliberate Instability

When you get out and play deliberately engage your core. Kettlebells and medicine balls are some of many tools you may use to work your core. Here is one other technique or point for consideration.

Balance and stability are key elements of our ability to move. Often in the gym, we focus on exercises that are smooth and clean moving through one plane of motion. In the gym we often operate on stable surfaces but life doesn't always present us with flat, smooth, stable surfaces. We rely most heavily on our core when we confront unstable surfaces.

The kettlebell, medicine balls, and other balls of all shapes and sizes can be used to create unstable surfaces.

CHAPTER 3 GET OUT & PLAY: THE CORE, BELLS & BALLS

Deliberately incorporate unstable surfaces into your play routines. This instability and testing of your balance will cause you to rely more deliberately on your core. The more you train your core, the better your posture will be, the stronger and more flexible your muscles and joints will be and the more fit you will become.

Balls of all shapes and sizes are tools for play. Use balls as tools to work your entire body but most specifically your core. A strong core is essential for overall fitness. A strong core will help reduce or eliminate back pain, sore necks and pulled muscles. A strong core is the key to a lifetime of mobility.

Work your whole body as you play every day and work it in a way to tax and train your core. A strong core is the basis for high performance fitness.

Ensure your play sessions challenge your core every day.

CHAPTER 4 MINDSET

Attitude Determines Altitude

Have you ever used a lever?

Sure you have.

You have used mechanical levers of all sorts your entire life. Levers allow us to move things. Even your body is made up of a number of levers. Muscles, bones and ligaments form levers in your body allowing you to move.

One of the capabilities of a lever is that it can provide a mechanical advantage. Using a lever we can move heavier loads than we could on our own. A renowned Greek mathematician, physicist, engineer, inventor and astronomer known as Archimedes once said, 'Give me a lever long enough and I can move the world.' Levers are powerful devices; devices which provide us potent advantages.

As we have seen, habits are our driving, routine actions. Habits ultimately determine our health and fitness. We choose our habits. We develop our habits. And we nurture and sustain our habits. But all habits are not equal.

Some habits have little impact and are of marginal consequence. Some habits however, are prime movers. These specific habits exert a disproportionate effect on the outcomes we enjoy or endure. Some habits wield a great deal of leverage. These powerful, far-reaching habits are "Lever Habits". Lever habits are the few key habits which matter most. Lever habits are tied to our core beliefs. Lever habits produce the results in life, good or bad, which we have grown accustomed to.

If you are approaching this high performance health and fitness change process in a deliberate way you have

CHAPTER 4 MINDSET: ATTITUDE DETERMINES ALTITUDE

probably conducted at least a cursory habits inventory. You have probably cataloged some good and some bad habits. The good news is you don't have to worry about changing every bad habit. You don't have to manage every detail of your transformation. To change yourself in a radical way all you must do is identify the few key lever habits setting you back.

To make a profound change in the course of your life adopt lever habits to take you in a new direction.

You have probably guessed: the lever habits that matter most regarding your overall health and fitness are your mindset, your nutrition and your play habits.

Here we draw back the curtain a little more to understand that real and lasting change requires we only get a few things right. Getting just a few things right affects core beliefs and leverages the habits process to engage our automatic pilot for optimum performance.

Mindset: Lever Habit #1

Lever habits are those habits which leverage the energy of life. Lever habits allow us to perform at our best. The most powerful lever habit of them all is mindset.

You have heard about the power of positive thinking. You are familiar with and perhaps even realize that having a positive attitude toward the task at hand, the circumstances and people you encounter, and toward life in general offers a distinct advantage. A positive attitude combined with a growth mindset separates the doers and achievers from all the rest. High performers nurture and deliberately cultivate the habit of employing a positive attitude and a growth mindset.

CHAPTER 4 MINDSET: ATTITUDE DETERMINES ALTITUDE

Airplane pilots understand to gain altitude, to climb to higher heights they must orient their planes wings a certain way toward the ground and toward prevailing wind currents. This orientation of the wings, of the plane in flight, is known as attitude. Flying high and straight and far is a matter of managing attitude. The plane's attitude determines the altitude the pilot flies. The same concept works for the rest of us, feet firmly on the ground. Our attitude determines our position in space; our ability to deal with the forces of gravity and prevailing winds. Our attitude determines how high we fly, how fast we travel and how far we go. Attitude determines altitude.

Healthy, fit people set themselves up for maximum performance by operating with a positive attitude.

To high performers life is an adventure full of opportunity and ripe with possibility. High performers hold onto and nurture core beliefs allowing them to learn, grow, advance and create.

For high performers, failure is not an option, not because high performers do everything well and succeed at everything they try, but because every attempt is a learning experience, an opportunity to grow.

High performers only accept good enough if it moves them on to something even greater. They are not content to just get by. High performers test their limits. High performers express their full potential. Once they set their sights on a goal, once they choose a course and determine a direction they always go the extra mile. If they can do better, if they have the time and energy to produce a better result, they will. Average is not satisfactory; exceptional is a high performer's standard.

CHAPTER 4 MINDSET: ATTITUDE DETERMINES ALTITUDE

A Positive Attitude and Growth Mindset

A positive attitude, growth mindset is a state of being creative, not competitive. The world offers an unlimited supply of resources and opportunity. The price to take advantage of the opportunities, to avail ourselves of the resources is to engage, to act. Positive attitude, growth mindset people; high performers; recognize this truth.

The world is not a place of lack; it's a place of abundance. High performers don't have to put anyone down to climb up. They don't have to beat someone out to get what they want. People with a positive attitude and growth mindset see the world as a playground. Obstacles are challenges to help them grow. They are properly grounded yet with an attitude which allows them to soar.

Don't get the wrong idea; high performers are not superhuman. These are people who have adopted habits which tip the balance in their favor. High performers maintain a positive attitude, growth mindset most of the time. Because they do, they are willing and able to advance. High performers are self-aware enough to recognize when they settle into a negative, fixed mindset. And they act to get out of that negative state as quickly as possible.

Sustaining a positive attitude and growth mindset in itself takes disciplined effort. A person with a positive attitude and growth mindset realizes that this journey of life is intimately dependent on the vehicle they are using to make the journey. Taking care of that vehicle; using it the right way, fueling it properly, supporting and guiding it for optimum performance; is not an afterthought. Proper care and maintenance of the vehicle is a requirement; it is and must be a habitual component of the journey. High performer knows they aren't going to get anywhere without

CHAPTER 4 MINDSET: ATTITUDE DETERMINES ALTITUDE

setting the conditions for health and fitness, vitality and wellbeing.

The lever habit of a positive attitude and growth mindset influences our awareness to take care of our bodies. A positive attitude and growth mindset causes us to recognize the need for getting enough rest and taking the time to recharge.

Maintaining a positive attitude and growth mindset requires feeding our minds with positive inspiration regularly and associating with positive, like-minded people as often as possible; the more often the better. Maintaining a positive attitude and growth mindset means focusing on worthwhile, creative tasks and setting challenging and achievable goals. Maintaining a positive attitude and growth mindset leads to building and sustaining a network of support; people to call on, collaborate with and rely on. No one succeeds alone. Maintaining health and fitness, vitality and wellbeing are much easier if we have a support network helping us along.

The Power of Thought

As we have suggested, thinking is perhaps a human beings most difficult and challenging undertaking. But thinking, thought, is the most powerful tool we have in our kit bag, our toolbox for life. Thought is the means to bridge the gap between the reality of circumstance, the world out there, and the potential, the supply of the unlimited source of this world and beyond. Building and maintaining an attitude and mindset that is in-synch with this reality, this high performance perspective means our core beliefs are:

All is right with the world.

I am safe and connected, competent and capable.

and

CHAPTER 4 MINDSET: ATTITUDE DETERMINES ALTITUDE

I have a purpose, a reason for being.

The preeminent lever to change your life; the quintessential high performance health and fitness habit; is cultivating a positive attitude and growth mindset.

People with positive attitudes are optimistic, confident, grateful people. They nurture a thankful disposition and cultivate a worthwhile and motivating vision. They have things to do, places to go, and people to see. The opportunity of life is now, why waste time? Optimistic, growth-oriented people realize life is not a sure thing. Sometimes they have to advance blindly. But they are willing to take risks. They embrace the challenge and relish the adventure.

Become a high performer with a positive attitude and growth mindset. Become a lifelong learner. By cultivating your mind you will prioritize properly fueling and maintaining your body. Take time daily to connect with your inner self and connect with others. You are immersed in the adventure, don't waste time. Focus your efforts intensely. Be goal oriented. And maintain a single-minded focus to accomplish your goals as quickly as possible.

Eliminate distractions, set worthwhile goals and persist. That is what this high performance health and fitness habits change process is all about. If you feel the method or process you employ is not correct, choose a new course. Just don't give up; keep moving forward. Vision and persistence are hallmarks of high performers; they are staples of a positive mindset. Go the extra mile to sustain and improve your health and fitness. Joyfully do what needs to be done. Do what average performers, the unhealthy and the unfit, refuse to do.

CHAPTER 4 MINDSET: ATTITUDE DETERMINES ALTITUDE

One Powerful Lever

A positive attitude and growth mindset is a force to use across all dimensions of life: physical, mental, emotional, spiritual, social, and material. A positive attitude and growth mindset allow opportunity and creativity to flow. With the right mindset you make the right choices, the smart choices to care for your body and improve your health and wellbeing.

A positive attitude and growth mindset are grounded in core beliefs. Remember though, if your beliefs aren't right now, you can begin to change course by taking new action, by developing new habits, by doing things differently. New habits produce new results, new results nurture new beliefs.

Once you believe you will see. Attitude determines altitude.

If your mindset is not right; if you are not performing up to your potential; if you are not making smart choices routinely, habitually, start small. Change one habit and then another. Aim for those lever habits. Once you are firmly in control of the levers life will begin anew. Tackle one habit after another until you tip the balance.

By changing your habits your attitude and mindset will change, your core beliefs will change and your performance will skyrocket. You will be fit and healthy, capable and skillful, and vitally alive.

CHAPTER 4 NUTRITION

Fat Is NOT the Enemy

Sometimes having the wrong information just doesn't matter. We can be misinformed and still live quite comfortably. Being mistaken about facts does not necessarily mean we won't be able to achieve our potential.

Believing certain erroneous concepts, ideas, notions or theories may not set us back at all. For instance until the sixteenth century and even for centuries after most people believed the world was flat. We might be able to think of a few relatively obscure ways believing the world was flat might have limited some, a very few people's lives, but for the most part believing the world was flat just didn't matter.

Transmitting information or communicating by means other than direct sight and sound was virtually inconceivable until Marconi invented the radio. Human flight and traveling beyond the confines of earth's atmosphere were once fantasies of science fiction and the stuff of vivid dreams and imaginings. Today we communicate instantaneously around the globe. Millions of people fly to far-off destinations every day. And mankind has sent probes to distant reaches of our galaxy and beyond. Sometimes we just don't grasp the big picture. We don't get our facts straight. We operate with misinformation. And sometimes these mistakes cost us dearly.

In this twenty-first century we rely on the wonders of science to serve us, protect us, move us and keep us fit and healthy. Tens of thousands of people all over the world are checking the facts, are trying to understand and explain how the world works. Tens of thousands of people set the conditions for us to make choices. Many of these choices

CHAPTER 4 NUTRITION: FAT IS NOT THE ENEMY

directly impact our own health and wellbeing and the health and wellbeing of those we love. Sometimes we just get it wrong.

A requirement of sustaining health and fitness is fueling our bodies with the right, the best fuels. We quite often and quite routinely take liberties with this requirement.

For the vast majority of people other factors come into play when establishing and sustaining nutrition habits. What we eat or what we put in our bodies might depend on what is most readily available. It might depend on what we can afford. What we consume or smoke might depend on how we feel emotionally. Or what we ingest might depend on who we are associating with and what we are after socially or psychologically. We don't always make the smart choices. We don't always make the best choices. We always have our reasons. Sometimes however, we make the wrong choices because we don't know any better. We are misinformed. We don't have our facts straight. Sometimes our health and fitness, our wellness and vitality suffer for it.

Health and fitness, proper or optimum nutrition is not a matter of conforming to a calorie equation: calories in versus calories out; energy units ingested versus energy units expended; how much we eat versus how much we do. The calorie equation is not the Holy Grail of health and fitness. Don't believe it is.

Here is another idea to let go of: fat is bad for us.

Fat Is NOT the Enemy

We embraced this idea that fat is bad for us by spreading misinformation, information which seemingly corresponds with logic. A single researcher drew a correlation between fat and weight gain, between consuming

CHAPTER 4 NUTRITION: FAT IS NOT THE ENEMY

fat and packing away fat. Through savvy marketing and passionate advocacy this researcher convinced the mainstream health and medical establishment of the voracity of his dubious findings. Once the spark caught fire all it took was for a little fanning of the flames and fat became public health enemy number one. We've got that wrong too.

The food, the nutrients we need to properly fuel and maintain our bodies; the nutrients we need to ensure our health and wellbeing are varied and complex. After all our bodies are complex, dynamic organisms; but we are living in an environment which provides everything we need; everything we need to get by and everything we need to excel. We individually and collectively must make the right choices. If we are to sustain good health we must develop good nutrition habits.

Peeling back the onion we realize we need hundreds of various inputs in various quantities to stay healthy. In terms of major categories however, we only need to know about a few: carbohydrates, fats and proteins. Carbohydrates, fats and proteins provide us calories and essential nutrients. Alcohol is a separate category. Don't be misled alcohol also contains calories. Calories are an energy unit, but to be healthy we need more than just energy. We need vitamins and minerals. We need water (pure water has no calories) and we need other nutritional aids like fiber and yeast, prebiotics and probiotics to ensure all aspects of our cooperative system flourish and thrive.

Fats, proteins and carbohydrates provide us energy. They are the means by which we consume vitamins and minerals and fiber and other trace elements to fuel and sustain our bodies and our being. By embracing the calorie myth and making fat public enemy number one we have turned society down a disease-ridden path.

CHAPTER 4 NUTRITION: FAT IS NOT THE ENEMY

There are some reasons, some very obvious reasons why the calorie and fat myths have continued to proliferate. Keeping the myths alive provides a number of benefits to wide swaths of the population. First, there is money to be made. Believing nutrition is all about providing calories the agricultural and food industries have gotten extremely good at delivering calories for little cost. The cost of growing, producing, processing, packaging and delivering calories has been on a steady decline for decades. We have ready access to more calories than we need, easily at a cost we can afford. Those calories just aren't in the right or best form for sustaining health and wellbeing. Where an opportunity to make money exists time, energy and attention focus and results ensue. Sometimes not the best results.

Every economic transaction has two beneficiaries. Money does not change hands unless two parties perceive an increase in value. While agricultural businesses, food and drink suppliers, medical, insurance and pharmaceutical companies and the politicians and bureaucrats in government all benefit by this system of delivering maximum calories at minimum cost the people who consume these calories receive a substantial, if less consequential or shall we say a rather ultimately harmful, benefit.

Calories the vast majority of Americans consume offer three main benefits: 1) The cost per energy unit is low (food is relatively cheap); 2) Food and drink are readily available (convenience, which is a factor of transportability and shelf-life, is a priority); and 3) The food and drink give us pleasure (they taste great). We, the consumers enjoy benefits under the current nutrition production and distribution system. What's not to love?

We absolutely need calories and we need vitamins and minerals and water and fiber and a host of other nutrients to

CHAPTER 4 NUTRITION: FAT IS NOT THE ENEMY

sustain health. But for our systems, our bodies to function optimally; to be healthy and fit; we need the right nutrients in the right measure at the right time. Nature has provided precisely what we need, in the right measure at the right time for thousands of years. It's only now that we have developed a system of highly processed food stuffs that we are undermining rather than advancing health.

As a tenet of nutrition we vilify fat and, except for a few notable outliers, we have whole-heartedly embraced carbohydrates as the lynchpin in our convenient, low-cost calorie distribution system. Of the three: fats, carbohydrates and proteins the one category of nutrients our bodies can get along without is carbohydrates. We malign fat and enthusiastically almost zealously pursue low fat diets, when we need, must have, and must consume fat to survive. While we champion carbohydrates as the elixir of youth our bodies can do just fine without carbohydrates at all. Does this make sense?

I am painting a picture that would seem to point to a simple resolution. Hold your horses. Changing course individually, if you have money and or time, access and information is easy. But reorienting a huge, complex system is a major task.

The Real Culprit

You've heard, "Too much of a good thing can be bad." The prime culprit in our twenty-first century nutritional distribution system debacle is sugar. Consuming sugar is what is throwing most Americans' bodies out of whack. Our bodies have not evolved to manage the copious amounts of simple sugars we consume in our drinks and in all the processed foods we consume. The simple answer for sustained health and wellbeing, the simple answer for our

CHAPTER 4 NUTRITION: FAT IS NOT THE ENEMY

long-term fitness and vitality are consuming fresh, whole, natural foods.

The body's systems evolved, and our automatic pilots are primed to operate on what is naturally available in our environment. We are connected to each other, to this planet and to what this planet produces naturally. To be fit and healthy, to engage our health and fitness automatic pilot choose and nurture habits providing fresh, whole, natural foods.

We must get off the convenient, low-cost, high calorie, high-sugar, processed food gravy train.

To improve health individually and put society on a course to health and wellbeing we must reverse course. Reversing course has huge economic implications. And nothing gets people's attention like money changing hands or an economy changing course. This is a hazardous trail to tread. Only our health and wellbeing, only the health and vitality of our nation and the world are at risk. Should we take the risk and change course?

Changing the food production and distribution system requires we address all types of second, third and fourth order effects. We have pilloried fat but we have gone to great lengths to devise, manufacture and distribute all kinds of fat substitutes. These fat substitutes, the most dangerous and debilitating of which are known as trans-fats, are used to improve the taste and texture of convenient, processed foods and extend shelf-life.

Also most of us have a sweet tooth. Simple sugars, in addition to appealing to our taste buds, are converted to energy within our bodies easily and directly. Simple sugars provide a quick pick-me-up. Since fat is the enemy and fat tastes good we have taken to increasing the amount of sugar

CHAPTER 4 NUTRITION: FAT IS NOT THE ENEMY

(and salt) to improve the flavor of processed foods. As a consequence, as a nation we have hooked ourselves on sugar. We are addicted to sugar.

Further complicating the nutrition supply system are pesticides and herbicides used on crops; antibiotics used to fatten livestock; and genetically modified organisms used for countless, mostly economic reasons.

We have, for the most part, destroyed our natural whole-food production and distribution system in favor of delivering low-cost, convenient, tasty, calorie units. Our system is broken. To respond, to navigate the labyrinth of this dysfunctional nutrition system we must first embrace the facts. We must learn the truth. Once armed with the truth we can start down a new path.

So What Then?

Habits drive our train. With the right habits we can go far and go fast. With the wrong habits we are going nowhere, we are headed for trouble. Change your nutrition, your eating habits.

First stop the madness, stop ingesting anything that might harm your body. Next start moving from a processed-foods based diet to a fresh, whole, natural-foods based diet.

To make this change you need not sacrifice taste. Changing from a traditional highly processed diet of convenience foods to a fresh, whole, natural-foods based diet need not cost you money. Making the change and developing a new habit however, is going to require your time, energy and attention. The results you get and the benefits you enjoy will be well worth it.

Here are a few tips to get you started. In later nutrition sections we will pursue these points in more detail:

CHAPTER 4 NUTRITION: FAT IS NOT THE ENEMY

1. Aim to eat only fresh, whole foods. Throw away or give away or get rid of anything with artificial sweeteners, trans-fats or high fructose corn syrup as an ingredient. Begin to trim back processed foods by counting the ingredients on the nutrition facts label. Aim to reduce the number of ingredients in the foods you buy. You will be successful when you only buy and consume foods without an ingredient label: whole, natural foods.

2. Shop the perimeter of the grocery store. The perimeter is where you find vegetables and fruits, meats, eggs and dairy products. Avoid the isles with highly processed foods. Avoid foods containing added sugar, sugar substitutes and added sodium.

3. Eat a salad every day. Consume a salad, preferably as your main meal once per day. Just by initiating this routine you are likely going to increase you vegetable intake and reduce your processed food consumption considerably.

Making even these changes are going to require time and effort. Learn about the foods you eat. What is in those packages? Find healthy substitutes to overcome urges you now have as you are likely addicted to sugar. Abandoning simple sugars, added sugars all together, will serve you well. Painstakingly, carefully and deliberately build new nutrition habits.

With the right nutrition habits you engage your automatic pilot appropriately. Your systems will operate as they should. Your body-chemistry will be in balance. You will be firing on all cylinders. You will be healthy.

It's all very simple really; it's just not necessarily easy.

Do it anyway.

CHAPTER 4 GET OUT AND PLAY

Body-Weight Play

Health and fitness is a multi-billion dollar industry. The field covers a large swath of everything from medicine to sports psychology to exercise physiology to meditation and acupuncture to nutrition and supplements to dieting and weight loss to gyms and exercise facilities and programs of all intensity levels, shapes and sizes. Go channel surfing at virtually any time of day or night and you will be besieged with a countless variety of must have gadgets and gizmos to help you become sleek and toned; strong and sexy, fit and healthy. Truth be told, you don't need all that stuff; you don't need any of that stuff. You don't need fancy gyms and pricey tools. You have everything you need, right here, right now, to get and keep yourself in tip top shape. Even the bells and the balls introduced earlier are not necessary.

All you need to improve and maintain fitness is a body, with moving parts, and some resistance. And guess what? The planet we are on just happens to supply, naturally, all the resistance we need. It's called gravity.

I'm not suggesting you cancel your gym membership; or throw away all those gadgets and gizmos. Gyms, classes, and programs provide much of the structure, discipline and social support we need to keep ourselves motivated, engaged and happy. Those gadgets and gizmos provide variety and keep things fresh and novel. Just remember, more important than all that stuff is actually doing something; taking action; playing every day.

In this OP section we focus quite literally on the tools you have at hand and the only tools you need to get and stay fit for life: your body and the resistance of gravity.

CHAPTER 4 GET OUT & PLAY: BODY-WEIGHT PLAY

In the Foreword I introduced the elements of fitness: body composition, cardiovascular endurance, muscular strength, muscular endurance, and flexibility. Fitness involves your entire body. We must properly warm up and stretch to begin any play session. In the last OP section we emphasized strengthening the core as your core is critical to stability, mobility, agility, power and strength. Here we focus on muscular strength and endurance.

Use Your Body-weight

Body-weight, weight-bearing exercises are movements to incorporate into every play session.

You have seen and executed an endless variety of body-weight exercises. Body-weight exercises are movements requiring you overcome the pull of gravity on your body. Overcoming the resistance of gravity conditions your body.

Our bodies have an amazing, adaptive capability. The more resistance we overcome, the more a body adapts to deal with the additional load or recurring resistance.

We are in an environment where, to survive and to thrive, we must overcome resistance. Our minds, our systems, our muscles and our organs adapt to the rigors of resistance we face. If we properly and appropriately subject our muscles and systems to stress, physical stress, not emotional or hormonal types of stress, our bodies automatically and naturally adapt. After repair, regeneration and rejuvenation we grow stronger and more capable. Overcoming resistance is an act of nature.

Where to start?

Let's start at the bottom, with our largest muscle groups; those in our legs and buttocks. Squats. I know,

CHAPTER 4 GET OUT & PLAY: BODY-WEIGHT PLAY

endless squats are not fun. Really though we squat all the time. We move like in a squat to stand up. We squat to reach down. We squat to lift things up.

Squats are a routine and common motion. We squat all the time. To be more comfortable moving around, to be more stable and more agile and more flexible incorporate squats deliberately and creatively into your daily play routine.

To squat properly maintain an erect posture; keep everything aligned; and bend at the knees and hips. Your knees should track out over your toes, but not extend beyond your toes. To maintain proper form you may have to sit back some. Squat down in a controlled, body-firm fashion and then power back up.

Try various types of squatting exercises: the standard two-legged squat, or if you are already pretty strong go to one-legged squats in any number of variations. Notice different people squat through different ranges of motion. The more squats you do, with increasing resistance and through larger ranges of motion, the stronger you will become. And don't fret; with diligent practice, over time, you will increase your range of motion.

A squat is an important component of a body fitness, a complete play program. Do what you can do, using good form. Determine to execute a number of squats that is a challenge to complete; always with good form. Then as you continue to build your play sessions, commit to doubling that number within a given time frame. Use your own body weight to strengthen your muscles.

The next lower body, body-weight exercise to incorporate in your play routine is the lunge. Again, you probably already know a variety of lunge movements. Here

CHAPTER 4 GET OUT & PLAY: BODY-WEIGHT PLAY

too form is key. If you are new to lunges, maintain a relatively small range of motion, but push yourself enough to feel the burn of resistance.

Squats and lunges put the muscles of your lower body to work. And like almost all exercises incorporate your core.

Moving Up

Next are two basic body weight movements to exercise your upper body: your chest, arms and shoulders, and your back.

The first upper body body-weight exercise is again a movement you are likely familiar with. This move is the essential component of a multitude of exercises. The most common body-weight variety is the push up. All you need is your body and the ground to push your weight against.

Try a number of push-up variants in a full plank position or on your knees: the standard, hands shoulder width or military style or hands wider than shoulder width placement. Try placing your hands at angles. Set yourself up on unbalanced or unstable surfaces. Elevate your feet. You can even suspend your body in the air. Push-up options are limited only by your imagination.

Settle on beginning with one version of the push-up you can do comfortably while maintaining proper form: body relatively straight. Determine how many repetitions of that version of a push-up you can do. Do push-ups, in some variety, every day during your play session. Set a goal and make it your mission to double that initial number of repetitions.

Doing a standard push-up, a push-up in a plank position, incorporates your core. Here again, form is important. Be careful not to stress your back. Do the style

CHAPTER 4 GET OUT & PLAY: BODY-WEIGHT PLAY

of push-ups you can do properly. Make the push-up part of your body-weight play session.

You probably can guess the next upper body, body-weight exercise. We just highlighted pushing against the resistance of gravity. Now we want to pull against the resistance of gravity. The pre-eminent pulling exercise is the pull-up or chin-up, again in a multitude of variants.

The pull-up uses muscles in the chest, shoulders, arms, back and core. If you can't do a single pull-up now, that is lift your own body to get your chin over a bar, make it your play session goal to strengthen your muscles enough to do a pull-up. Oh, and women can do pull-ups. It comes down to deliberately, consistently overcoming resistance.

Two things make pull-ups and push-ups, squats and lunges, and all other body movements easier. The first thing is strong, fit muscles; the second is no excess body weight.

Save Time, Play Hard

As you develop your play session consider incorporating what may be the most power-packed, time condensed method of play. Using this technique you can complete an entire session of body-weight exercises in as little as ten minutes.

Rather than struggling to push or pull your weight up focus on resisting as gravity naturally pulls your body down. This is known as eccentric movements.

Eccentric exercises focus on slowing down the elongation portion of a muscle movement after a contraction. You contract the muscle while lengthening it at the same time. For instance in a squat rather than focusing on the standing up phase of the squat focus on slowly settling down. You can do this with two legs, but to increase the intensity,

CHAPTER 4 GET OUT & PLAY: BODY-WEIGHT PLAY

the amount of work your muscles accomplish, try resisting gravity's pull while slowly squatting on one leg. Work both legs until you can execute a sequence of eccentric movements comfortably then move to one leg alone.

The crux of the eccentric motion in a squat is delaying, slowing down your descent. Sink into the squat slowly through a ten-count. If you are able to do six or more repetitions with perfect form using both legs, move to single leg squats. Focus on the eccentric phase, a ten-count down, and then use both legs to stand back up. Repeat the exercise for a minimum of six repetitions on each leg.

To build stronger muscles, to improve muscle repair and to increase your metabolic rate focus on the eccentric phase of these low-impact body-weight exercises.

Six eccentric squats per leg.

Execute a minimum of six lunges on each leg. Concentrate on the eccentric phase, slowly lower your weight through a ten-count.

Execute the eccentric motion on a push-up. Here too you can increase resistance on each arm. To put more resistance on one arm at a time, after pushing up with both arms shift your weight over the one arm you are training. Use your other arm for balance only while you lower your body weight for a ten-count. Again do at least six repetitions with each arm.

Execute the eccentric motion on a pull up. Pull yourself up, leg-assisted if necessary, and then slowly lower yourself down for a ten-count. Complete two sets of six repetitions for maximum results.

Eccentric exercises, particularly those done at maximum effort may produce the best strength gains and

CHAPTER 4 GET OUT & PLAY: BODY-WEIGHT PLAY

initiate the most beneficial metabolic triggers for the least amount of time committed.

As you grow stronger add more resistance to these moves with weights or weighted vests or straps and bands and so on. Just remember, ultimately strengthening your body is all about overcoming resistance. When you overcome resistance deliberately and intelligently your body responds.

To be a high performer; to be healthy and fit; let your body achieve its potential. Develop a positive attitude and growth mindset. Provide your body with the optimum fuel. And present the necessary resistance in the right measure and in the right doses. When you do; you are on the road to high performance health and fitness.

Once on the right road your automatic pilot kicks in. You will automatically shed excess pounds, firm and strengthen muscles, and increase the capacity of all your physiological systems.

You have everything you need to play and play well. You have a body and you have gravity. Put your body to the test; make a habit of overcoming resistance every day.

The more you do the stronger and more capable you become.

CHAPTER 5 MINDSET

How To

The most wonderful, extraordinary and absolutely terrifying thing about life is that we are immersed in this action-adventure, drama, comedy, tragedy, and love story. We are completely submerged in and engrossed with this reality. We get to see it, taste it, hear it, smell it, and most of all feel it. More than that we get to analyze it, assess it, and choose to absorb or reject what we experience. Even more than that we get to write and direct; we choose our course. We conceive and create in the epic. This truly is a magnificent journey, an awesome opportunity.

The two simplest evocative words I can think of to describe the unique experience of this adventure called life are "feel" and "act". Immersed in this adventure we absorb energy and we interpret what we experience through feelings. We feel life. We feel the adventure, good and bad. More than watching a movie or even a live performance on stage we experience life through what we feel.

And we act. A uniquely remarkable benefit of life is we get to move. We are actors, expressing life. The energy of life flows through us as we move within this complex and beautiful environment. This is truly an astonishing and astounding journey.

Life is a "feeling–action" process. We feel and we act. Feelings motivate us, they move us to act. Some people act more and move more, and some act less and move less. But all of us move and all of us act. Within the energy flow of life change happening about us is happening within us and is happening to us. There is no avoiding it. We are riding the wave of life. We chose to be here. We have traveled to

CHAPTER 5 MINDSET: HOW TO

where we are. The opportunity is we get to choose where to go next.

Life is like a game show. We are always picking the magic door. We are always searching for and anticipating the next prize. Let's make a deal.

Life is a Feeling-Action Process

Everyone wants to be happy. "Happy" however, is a loaded word. We often attach all kinds of conditions to what "happy" means. For some those conditions are achievement, wealth and possessions, respect and esteem, love and acceptance. Rather than wrestle with conditions let's simply define "happy" this way: We are happy when we feel good physically, emotionally, intellectually, and spiritually. We are happy when we feel, deep within our beings, connected, capable, secure and joyful. Happiness doesn't depend one iota on external circumstances or on our environment and our situation. Happiness is a state of acceptance and joy; a state we choose to embrace; a state we are free to move into anytime.

To be happy you don't have to be at your best emotionally or physically. You don't even have to be healthy. This body you have been given, this body you occupy is your ally, it's your partner, it's your collaborator on this journey of life. Your body is not meant to be a hindrance. You are truly meant to be happy. Every day of this life, every moment of this life you have an opportunity to choose happiness. Your body means to help you realize what you want to achieve in this life. Your body comes with an automatic pilot to keep your systems working as they should. Your body intends to help you feel good and to allow you to feel happy. But setting the conditions for your body to do what comes naturally, to do what it is meant to do

CHAPTER 5 MINDSET: HOW TO

automatically, requires you properly guide and support. You must take care of yourself.

We are much more likely to feel happy if we are operating on all cylinders; if our physiological systems are functioning optimally. This means we must choose, adopt and nurture the right habits.

A habit is a routine response to a given stimulus; a process moving us from craving to reward by way of action. Life is a feeling–action process. Make this process work for you.

Habits are powerful tools because habits leverage feelings to keep us moving in a specific direction. Build the right habits, habits which empower and ensure success. The million dollar question is: How?

Why?

How do we develop and nurture the right habits; mindset habits, nutrition habits and play habits; to reach and enjoy our full potential?

The "how to" is simple, but not easy.

We prefer to jump straight to the "how to". We all want to know how to succeed and get rich. We all want to know how to find love and joy and be happy. We think the "how to" is the answer. The "how to" is not the answer.

Let's clarify: the "how to" comes into play but only down the road. The "how to" matters only after we settle on and determined "why". "Why" is our motivation. "Why" rests in how we feel. "Why" nests with core beliefs.

Why do you want to be healthy and fit? Why do you want to look and feel better? Why do you want to be leaner and more powerful, more skillful and more capable? If you

CHAPTER 5 MINDSET: HOW TO

have a powerful enough "why", a powerful enough reason, a powerful enough motivation, you will begin to change your feeling–action process. A powerful "why" moves you to act in a new way.

If you really want to change you will change. It's a choice. But you must want to make that choice. You must want to change. Feelings of desire must be greater than feelings of resistance. If your desire is strong enough you can overcome any challenge. You have what you need to go where you want to go. The choice of where to go and what to become is up to you.

When you are ready, when you are motivated to change course the "how to" will help you proceed.

The remainder of this section focuses on the "how to". In Appendix B is a step by step process for changing habits. This habits change process applies to all habits not just health and fitness habits. Execute that "how to" process to change the simplest of habits and to acquire and develop powerful lever habits. But first be clear on "why".

The Habits Change Process

In an earlier section we explored two approaches to life:

First, the approach we use for new or unfamiliar circumstances. This approach is the one we rationalize as being our primary means of dealing with circumstances (we like to think we are both rational and thoughtful):

STIMULUS > FEELING > THOUGHT > ACTION > REWARD

Second, is the approach we use most of the time:

CHAPTER 5 MINDSET: HOW TO

STIMULUS > FEELING > ACTION > REWARD – THOUGHT (if needed)

We develop and rely on habits, our energy conservation devices, most of the time.

A habit cycle is composed of four parts:

1) The stimulus, situation or circumstance which

2) Triggers a feeling, desire or craving which

3) Initiates a routine act or action which

4) Achieves a reward or provides resolution.

A habit cycle is automatic, no thinking required.

The first step in how to change your habits is to determine exactly what habits are dominating your life now. Conduct a habits inventory. Over the course of a week (you may enlist some trusted allies to help you with this) assess and catalog all the things you do habitually. This will require real concentration and genuine self-awareness.

Get yourself a notebook and keep it handy. Build a list of everything you do every day habitually. Once you note a habit the first time, just keep count the rest of the week on how many times you repeat that sequence. To help wipe away clutter and keep yourself focused specifically on health and fitness habits pay particular attention to how you respond to hunger, stress and other emotional cues which move you to consume something. And carefully catalog you play, activity or exercise routines.

Construct a list of habits related to what you put in your body, how you treat your body and what you do with your body. Health and fitness is a total being effort, an effort

CHAPTER 5 MINDSET: HOW TO

involving your biology, psychology, spirituality and social connections, but for now, to keep things simple, examine most closely nutrition and play habits.

At the end of the week review your list. How is your "habits ratio": good nutrition and play habits relative to bad?

If your inventory is dominated by bad habits don't be discouraged. You have gotten to where you are incrementally, gradually over time. Don't expect overnight results, but by moving in a new direction you can expect steady progress.

Work on one habit at a time. Replace bad habits, habits which don't serve you, with good habits, habits which move you forward. You never totally eliminate a bad habit routine from your psyche. That habit routine will always be with you, so you are at risk of falling back. Be ready for that. Taking a step back is not failure. Don't ever give up; keep moving forward.

Choose one bad habit to replace. Keep it simple; perhaps a snacking routine. Aim ultimately to adopt high performance lever habits (positive attitude, growth mindset; proper nutrition and play habits) but don't overreach at the start.

Begin to see from a new perspective. Begin changing what you believe. To do that, change what you experience. Implement new habit routines and faith will grow. Soon a new good habit will take the place of that bad habit.

Refer to Appendix B for the specific *Habits Change Process* steps.

Step by step, habit by habit create a whole new you.

CHAPTER 5 MINDSET: HOW TO

How to do it; how to change course, how to adopt new habits is not nearly as important as actually doing something; moving in a new direction.

If your motivation to change is weak focus your efforts on developing your "why" then turn to the "how to".

You can change; it's within your power; but you must want to change. If you are motivated enough the "how to" will evolve naturally.

Even small steps, if you keep taking them, will take you very far. Keep moving forward.

CHAPTER 5 NUTRITION

Diet and Exercise

If you don't feel great, if you don't think you look great, if you are overweight or out of shape you have probably tried "conventional wisdom" any number of times. Conventional wisdom tells us: in order to lose weight and get fit reduce our calorie intake and increase our calorie output. Conventional wisdom tells us quite definitively that health and fitness are all about diet and exercise.

Well conventional wisdom is correct to a degree, but only if we properly define our terms. When most of us think of diet, diets or dieting, we don't think about our standard, long-term, routine of nutrition; our eating habits. Diets or dieting usually means sacrifice and cutting back for a relatively short period of time. The party is over and deprivation begins. We diet when it's time to get serious. We elect to start starving ourselves. And we get on the treadmill and begin the trudge to nowhere.

Diets do work. Diets in the traditional, conventional wisdom sense work. Cutting back calories causes pounds to drop. But dieting, in the traditional "cutting back" sense, rarely makes us healthy and fit.

If we put out more calories than we take in our bodies realize something is out of the ordinary and adjusts. Remember we are really part of a cooperative and this cooperative functions by certain rules.

As our body's main concern is survival, recognizing a calorie deficit the body shifts to conservation mode. Initially the body attempts to conserve calories from inputs and store them as fat. If physical activity (that endless treadmill) demands calories beyond what are readily available the body

CHAPTER 5 NUTRITION: DIET AND EXERCISE

reprioritizes the calorie draw. First it uses up energy in the blood. As glucose levels fall the body triggers all kinds of cravings for simple sugars and sweets; easy energy. If those cravings don't do the trick (will power is usually strongest at the beginning of a diet) the body will begin to draw down stores. Protein from muscle will typically be thrown into the fire before fat. Burning fat is a last resort.

If a person starves themselves, following the convention wisdom of dieting, once fat starts burning the body is going pull out all the stops. Metabolism is going to slow, cravings are going to skyrocket and the battle of wills will be joined.

The average attempt at dieting lasts about 14 days. Dieting is typically a battle of wills. We try to outsmart and outmaneuver our bodies. We think we can circumvent or at least temporarily override our habits process. Even though virtually any diet that reduces calories-in relative to calories-out will shed pounds, we rarely hang in. We just can't hang on. Will power is a finite resource. We fight a losing battle. Not a battle of losing weight, rather a losing battle against ourselves.

For those who do endure, those successful dieters who lose weight most are not able to keep the weight off. They typically pack the pounds back on. You have heard of yoyo dieting. We engage in the battle of wills. We take it off. We let our guards down. We fall into old habit patterns. We put the weight back on again and usually add a little more as the body now has to prepare for future bouts with starvation. Conventional wisdom, diet and exercise, does not go far enough.

We must change our eating habits. Really we must change our mindsets, our nutrition habits and our play habits

CHAPTER 5 NUTRITION: DIET AND EXERCISE

if to be healthy and fit and to stay that way. Dieting is too often a "one-time" or "some-time" thing; something we engage in when things have gone from bad to worse; when we're desperate. Dieting, those crash diets or fad diets, is not the answer.

Changing your lifestyle, changing your habits is the answer.

The Right Diet

So just what does dieting mean nutritionally?

Have you heard of or attempted any of these diets?

Cookie diet	South Beach diet	Subway diet
Scarsdale diet	Beverly Hills diet	Grapefruit diet
Hacker's diet	Cabbage soup diet	Juice Fast diet
Liquid diet	Swank diet	Warrior diet

How about, have you signed on to any of these program diets?

Jenny Craig	Weight Watchers	Nutrisystems

Or have you attempted or adopted a life-style diet?

Kosher diet	Islamic halal diet	Vegetarian diet
Lacot-ovo Vegetarian diet		Vegan diet
Low fat diet	Eat-clean diet	Gluten free diet
Low sodium diet	Low glycemic index diet	
Low carbohydrate diet	High protein diet	
Ketogenic diet (high fat, low-carb)		Fit for Life diet

CHAPTER 5 NUTRITION: DIET AND EXERCISE

And this is only the tip of the iceberg. You can probably come up with another dozen diets without even putting much effort into it.

Some people choose a nutrition path conforming to their values. The majority of health conscious Americans temporarily follow specific diet guidelines. Most people settle onto a nutrition path out of convenience or necessity. With a myriad of options, we are left to consider: Which diet is the best? And which one is right for me?

These questions don't have easy specific answers because everyone is different and everyone sees the world from a different perspective and everyone has a slightly different value set. In general terms however, the answer is simple. Eat foods which optimize the functioning of your body and physiological systems and eat foods which vitalize and energize you.

That answer doesn't really give you much help. The truth is you have to find the answer for yourself. But here is where to start.

Remember the key is developing and nurturing life-enhancing nutrition habits. Once you have the right eating habits your body's automatic pilot takes control and your system will function as well as it possibly can.

The fundamentals of sound eating habits and a good diet are: eat fresh, whole, organic or natural foods and drink plenty of water. The details beyond that are up to you to work out. But start here:

Check out these diets, these life-style eating systems, and begin to build your own helpful, life-enhancing, vitalizing eating habits:

DASH diet

CHAPTER 5 NUTRITION: DIET AND EXERCISE

Atkins diet

Mediterranean diet

Paleo diet

What you find in common between these diets and with any nutritionally sound dietary system is an emphasis on fresh, whole, natural foods. All of these diets call for the elimination or at least radical reduction of processed foods, artificial sweeteners and artificial ingredients of any kind. These diets intend to eliminate or reduce to the greatest degree possible pesticides and agricultural chemicals, the consuming of any food stuffs grown or raised dependent on the administration of antibiotics, chemicals or drugs, and the consumption, directly or indirectly of genetically modified organisms.

Fresh, whole, natural, organic foods and clean, clear water and green tea provide the nutrients to properly fuel our bodies. Change your habits to consume fresh, whole, natural foods instead of the typical American diet; what is commonly known as the fast-food or junk-food diet.

The American food production and distribution system, driven primarily by agri-business, pharmaceutical interests, and the components of government these entities control, is built upon quantity and convenience over quality and health. The system provides highly processed (for ease of transportation and long shelf-life), high-calorie options conveniently available for relatively low cost.

Consumers want food stuffs which are easy to acquire and pleasurable to eat. We want tasty, cheap food fast. The system provides just that. It is a remarkable system really, but it is not the best system for promoting health and wellbeing.

CHAPTER 5 NUTRITION: DIET AND EXERCISE

Americans are masters at achieving what we set our minds to. We have a system where we get lots of calories at little cost. To be healthy and fit, break with the system. Do not subscribe to the great American diet. Make smarter choices about what you put in your body.

Fresh, whole, natural foods are the way to go. Remember, consume protein and consume fat. Consume vitamins and minerals and fiber and probiotics (good bugs for your gut) but you don't need carbs. We are eating and drinking heavily processed foodstuffs made with artificial ingredients and with all kinds of added sugars. Our food supply is killing us. Be a radical; choose a different approach.

You and I can't change the system however we can be voices for change. We don't have the luxury of time to wait for "the system" to get it right. Make the right choices, the smart choices now. And make those choices habits.

To make the right choice you need viable options and you need the right information. Once you have both set yourself up to adopt the best nutrition habits. Eat only fresh, whole, natural foods.

If you are ready to dig into the details see the **Recommended Reading** list in the back of this book (Appendix C). That list is only three books long. This is a great starting place to dig into the details. Figure out which food stuffs are best, are right for you. Then develop habits taking thought out of your nutrition equation. You will be on the path of long-term health and fitness.

CHAPTER 5 GET OUT AND PLAY

Yoga and Pilates

Once again it is time to play. Maybe you can venture outside to breathe in fresh air and to absorb warming rays of sunshine. Go out to escape all those electronic distractions strategically placed around the house to keep us connected, entertained and ultimately stressed.

In this section we briefly cover two disciplines. Discipline is a good word for these practices. These disciplines are systems for the development of mind and body: Yoga and Pilates.

I bring these two up together, yoga and Pilates; because they are both low impact practices emphasizing proper breathing, range of motion, and body control.

Yoga is thousands of years old. The word "yoga" originated literally from the concept of yoking oxen together. Yoga is a discipline of mind, body and spirit intended to optimize both how the practitioner feels and how the practitioner experiences life. Yoga is a deliberate practice of binding yourself to free yourself.

Pilates, on the other hand, is a relatively new development. Joseph Pilates studied both Eastern and Western forms of exercise and developed, in the 1930's and '40's, a system intended to strengthen both the mind and body. One of the main differences between yoga and Pilates is the use, in Pilates, of various apparatus. These apparatus, or devices, are designed to speed the process of strengthening, lengthening and aligning the body and increasing core strength begun by work on the mat.

CHAPTER 5 GET OUT & PLAY: YOGA AND PILATES

Over the years, and for yoga that's over millennia, both yoga and Pilates have evolved. Various schools and devotees have focused on several aspects of these practices and have combined them with other exercises and practices in a countless assortment of ways.

If you were to go to two different yoga or Pilates studios, studios not owned and operated under the same management umbrella, you are likely to find different and distinct practices and methods. The studios will execute common movements, but you will also likely find some distinctive features. Variety is the spice of life. So don't sweat the differences, embrace them. Incorporate what works best for you and discard the rest. Do the best you can with what you have. You can't do more than that; and that's good enough for maintaining your health and fitness.

We are not going to concern ourselves with or get lost in the details. These are valuable tactics, techniques, and procedures; valuable practices and exercises to incorporate regularly into your play routines. Both yoga and Pilates are worthwhile health and fitness practices.

Yoga

As we have emphasized right from the beginning of this program breathing is an essential component of health and fitness. Incorporating beneficial breathing practices will help you get and stay healthy and fit. Breathing is a systems activity. You need the vital nutrients of the air, the energy of the environment to function, to live. We are connected, integrated into this environment through the process of breathing. Yoga is one of the best methods for learning to breathe properly.

Yoga is a low impact type of activity. But, don't let that fool you. Most men, especially the "he-men want-to-

CHAPTER 5 GET OUT & PLAY: YOGA AND PILATES

be's" avoid yoga because they think it's a delicate practice meant for the fairer of the sexes. Don't kid yourself. Yoga will help you with all aspects of fitness: body composition, flexibility, strength, and endurance. Yoga helps clear your mind and helps relieve stress. The benefits of yoga are endless and reach into all aspects of life. Don't judge; try it. I bet you will find yoga challenging and relaxing, perhaps even liberating.

Yoga is a diverse and evolved practice. You will find all types of environments and systems for practicing yoga. The main elements are: first, controlling your breathing, and second, fluid body movement through deliberate ranges of motion. These ranges of motion incorporate a number of body-weight exercises or poses and postures.

Each of these poses or postures has a name. Often yoga routines advance through poses and postures in deliberate sequences. The poses engage, stretch and work all your muscles. You move deliberately all while controlling your breathing.

These movements, this body-weight work, through these postures will get your blood flowing. You will sweat when practicing yoga. You don't have to sweat, and you could focus more on the meditative aspect of yoga and that's a good thing too. But you can work all your muscles, and exercise most of your bodily systems practicing yoga.

The third component of yoga is balance. Some of us have a hard enough time just standing still on our own two feet. I've been there. Yoga will move you to balance in a squat, in a lunge, with hands held high, with hands extended to the side. You will balance on one foot and one hand. You will balance on one foot by itself and balance on your hands. You get the picture.

CHAPTER 5 GET OUT & PLAY: YOGA AND PILATES

Yoga is a complete mind-body system of play focusing on proper breathing, moving through a wide range of motion and balance. You would be hard-pressed to find a more comprehensive and ultimately refreshing and liberating play system for overall health and fitness. Try out different yoga classes and studios. Try different instructors and different styles of yoga until you find the perfect fit.

Yoga could be your everyday play routine. At a minimum however, consider incorporating yoga into your overall health and fitness program once per week. The benefits will add up.

Pilates

With Pilates there is, or can be a lot of mat work. In addition or instead you might work extensively with select, specially designed apparatus. Students of Joseph Pilates defined six principles which have since become widely accepted amongst Pilate's practitioners as the core elements of the program. These six principles are: Concentration; Control; Centering; Flow or efficiency of movement; Precision; and Breathing.

Pilates, like any beneficial play, requires focus and concentration. Every movement flows from precise breathing and by engaging the core. Like yoga, Pilates utilizes controlled, precise movements flowing in sequence. A correct, proper movement delivers much more benefit than an incorrect or half-hearted movement.

Joseph Pilates, after much research, testing and experimentation, ended up focusing on more aggressive styles of breathing than those typically found in yoga. He incorporated a more forceful breathing technique into his Pilates exercise program. The idea is to get more fresh air flowing through your system as we rely on the nutrients, the

CHAPTER 5 GET OUT & PLAY: YOGA AND PILATES

energy of air, to live and move. To get more good air in, you have to get the bad or used-up air out. Pilates employs pulsing exercises to synchronize body motion with forced inhalations or exhalations to optimize air flow.

In Pilates much can be done on the mat and much can be done using specialized apparatus. As for work on various apparatus, Pilates will force you to hurdle flexibility and range of motion roadblocks. Hurdle may be too aggressive a word to appropriately describe what you will do. Just know flexibility and range of motion are elements Pilates practice emphasizes. Pilates engages muscles, certain muscles not normally engaged as directly or as forcefully except through the use of specialized apparatus. Pilates is a well thought out; well defined system.

Find the Right Fit

Look for an instructor, whether for yoga or Pilates, who knows his or her stuff. If you get the right instructor, a teacher and coach you connect with, one who nurtures your progress in the right way and in the right environment, you can't go wrong with yoga or Pilates.

Give yoga and Pilates a try. Incorporate these practices into your play routines. Make a habit of yoga and Pilates; perhaps one session per week.

Either one, yoga or Pilates or both, could become and serve as the cornerstone of your play regimen. Yoga and Pilates are low-impact physical and mental practices integrating all body movement aspects of developing and maintaining health and well-being.

Yoga and Pilates are two more worthwhile forms of play to make you stronger, improve your fitness and ensure your long-term health.

CHAPTER 6 MINDSET

The Straw that Broke the Camel's Back

Life is filled with stress. We explore and experience, learn and grow, create and contribute in a stressful environment. To do anything at all we must deal with stress and overcome resistance.

Everything about life is in motion. Everything is constantly changing. As we navigate a course through constant change we feel energy flow. We also feel resistance. Sometimes we synchronize our motion with certain forces, energy in motion, and move in the same direction. Sometimes we oppose certain forces and work at odds with energy in motion. This "energy in motion" is resistance.

The resistance we face in the environment, from gravity to wind to water to heat and cold to the mechanical resistance of matter to the resistance we feel in our bodies from weakness to illness to disease to malfunction to the resistance we struggle with in our minds from confusion to anxiety to laziness to pride to fear are all natural elements of this reality. All the resistance in the environment around us, in our bodies and in our minds, is resistance we are challenged to face and must face.

Life is not easy. We are here to do something, something of consequence, something extraordinary. We are involved in something difficult and challenging and wonderful. The challenges we face, the obstacles we conquer, the resistance we overcome are our lessons, our means to growth. By overcoming resistance we change our perspective and we gain experience, first to reveal our potential and then to achieve it.

CHAPTER 6 MINDSET: THE STRAW THAT BROKE THE CAMEL'S BACK

Life, a Whole Lot of Stress, a Whole Lot of Wonderful

You are familiar with the adage, "The straw that broke the camel's back." Thinking about a single piece of straw it's difficult to imagine a single straw breaking a camel's back. One single straw is light and flexible; it weighs hardly anything at all. But under a load, under a heavy load, the addition of one piece of straw, only one light piece of straw, will serve as the measure that goes too far. It will be the straw that breaks the camel's back. The addition of that one small measure of weight, the addition of that one small measure of resistance is the final measure of stress which breaches the tipping point and causes the cataclysmic event: breaking the camel's back.

We human beings operate best in a range. We are intimately connected to the environment. We need air to breathe. We need water to drink and food to eat. We must maintain our body at a certain temperature, neither too hot nor too cold. We require a certain amount of air pressure as well, not too much or too little to function optimally or to function at all. To live requires just the right setting with just the right balance, the right range of conditions.

We, body and mind, are well equipped to deal with, manage and overcome stress. We, body, mind and spirit, have entered into a world with the purpose of dealing with stress, of managing stress and of overcoming stress. But there is a point where stress can be too much; a point where we take on too much or we produce too much; a point where stress overcomes and overwhelms us.

Stress can be a positive motivation to change and a positive means for growth or it can be an insidious force wearing us down and ultimately destroying us. To be

CHAPTER 6 MINDSET: THE STRAW THAT BROKE THE CAMEL'S BACK

healthy and fit, to be vitally alive, to go as far as we can as fast as we can on this journey of life we must carefully manage stress. We must keep ourselves in that optimum range, in the productive zone. While too little stress can be a bad thing, too much stress can be dangerous.

Stress comes in many forms. Stress demands some of our energy: some of our time and some of our attention. If we let it, stress will take some of our life.

We are playing on a vast and magnificent playground. We are on the adventure of a lifetime. We must be cautious though. We are not the biggest players on the playground. We must understand our limits, what we can and cannot do. And we must know how much stress we need to grow and advance and how much we can withstand to keep from being set back.

We are familiar with stressors in the environment; things like gravity and air and water and wind and weather. Collectively we have learned to mitigate many, if not most of the effects of nature. We heat the cold and cool the heat. We shelter ourselves from wind and water. We use the forces of gravity to refashion the environment we occupy. Not that we have conquered nature and nature's forces, but we recognize and for the most part deal with those forces effectively.

Other types of stress however, test us. We have mentioned the laws of motion before. A body at rest tends to stay at rest, while a body in motion tends to stay in motion. To cause something to change direction, speed up or slow down, requires an intervening force. We encounter those forces all over the external environment, but we encounter those forces within ourselves as well.

CHAPTER 6 MINDSET: THE STRAW THAT BROKE THE CAMEL'S BACK

Clearly we see that falling off a cliff is not likely to end well. The force of gravity is going to cause a cataclysmic event in a single instant. Too much stress will generate a significant change. But while we must be vigilant against environmental threats, physical forces, it's the forces we don't see so clearly which pose the most significant threats.

We face biological threats, pathogens and toxins, bacteria and viruses, threats to the functioning of our bodies. We human beings are social animals. We have needs and desires to bond, to be together, to love and be loved. These social needs are a prevalent source of stress; some good and some bad. And of course within our own psyches is a wellspring of potential stressors, the most notable and insidious of which is fear.

Manage Stress

To become and to be healthy and fit, to become and to be vitally alive effectively manage stress. Stress manifests in the environment, in our bodies and in our minds. Learn to manage stress in all its forms and in all its manifestations. Develop habits to mitigate stress and keep your mind and body operating in the optimal range.

Don't take on that straw, that one straw which initiates the cataclysmic event.

Deal with physical stress, social stress, biological and physiological stress and psychological stress. Use the very same strategy to deal with stress as to change health and fitness. Develop habits to routinely and automatically address stress.

Explore different habit strategies to manage stress. Include mind and body practices like meditation and prayer,

CHAPTER 6 MINDSET: THE STRAW THAT BROKE THE CAMEL'S BACK

yoga and martial arts. Or attempt a more deliberate approach to comedy and humor and joy-filled play.

Take time to consider all the stressors in your life. Carefully look beyond environmental stressors and examine the biological, social, and personally psychological sources of stress. Examine how you habitually respond to these stressors. Do certain stressors empower performance? Do certain stressors make you weak or ill?

Can you recognize certain stressors working in tandem setting you back?

Then consider your habitual responses to stress. Examine specifically the forces not serving to energize and move you forward. These stressors drain you; they demand your energy.

Is your habitual response to stress to attempt to power through?

Or do you absorb too much stress, collapse and then regroup to recover and recuperate?

Or do you ignore the stress and the toll stress is exacting on your mind and body over time?

None of these are winning strategies. You already have what you need to succeed. You have what you need to address stress too. You just have to engage and employ your assets.

Put your habits process to use. Adopt and nurture habits to mitigate stress automatically. Factor stress predominantly in your habits change process equation. Stress can motivate or stress can harm. Stress influences you in obvious and not so obvious ways.

CHAPTER 6 MINDSET: THE STRAW THAT BROKE THE CAMEL'S BACK

Lever habits serve naturally as stress mitigation and stress reduction tools. If your mind is right, if you believe in yourself, that is, you have faith in this world and you have a purpose for being, you approach life with a positive attitude and growth mindset. If you are taking care of your body; fueling your body properly, getting enough rest and enough quality sleep (at least eight hours per night); and if you are engaging joyfully in play at every opportunity you will control stress.

Stress is part of life. The stressors of life make us who we are. But too much stress is a bad thing. Too much stress from all sources or from any one source can be the straw to break our will. Develop habits of mind and habits of action to put you on a road to "stress-free living".

Be mindful of the straw; the little stressors in your life. Get out in front of potential stressors and take charge. To successfully navigate life you must go through the middle. Some things will scare you; some things will be bigger and more powerful than you. Some things will set you back. That's just the way it is. Don't let avoidable stress and stress you generate be that thing.

Be mindful of the straw and keep yourself from stressing out.

CHAPTER 6 NUTRITION

One Step at a Time

You have probably dieted before. You have probably made plans to eat healthy before. You have attempted to change course. What might be different this time? How can you actually make a change big enough and consistent enough to put you permanently on a path to health and wellbeing, fitness and vitality?

You are already moving; marching through life. You can't call a time-out. You can't halt the motion or stop the constant movement. You can however, manage your direction and speed. You set the course. You set the pace. Not everything is under your control but you have the power, the energy, and the insight you need to make smart choices, to make the right choices.

Change by taking one step at a time in a new direction.

Changing Eating Habits

You are already somewhat familiar with the "Habits Change Process". You have reviewed the process in an earlier chapter and you can follow the process as annotated in the appendix.

The main difference between this change process and most dieting and exercise programs is that in *High Performance Health and Fitness Habits* we do not focus on food and nutrition formulas (calories and ratios of nutrients, etc.) and specific exercises and activities as much as we focus on habits and what comes naturally.

Your body is designed for optimum performance. Your body will adapt both to its environment, current conditions, and the fuel it is provided. If the environment,

CHAPTER 6 NUTRITION: ONE STEP AT A TIME

conditions and fuel are optimal the body will automatically take care of the details. Health and fitness are automatic. If any of these, the environment, conditions, or the fuel supply are less than optimal the body will make modifications. We get what we get.

The process for making real and lasting change initially requires thought and reflection. You must pick a direction. Then take thought out of the equation and set yourself on automatic pilot.

You have developed your current eating habits over the course of your lifetime. Choosing a new course is simple. Empowering yourself with new habits is not so easy.

Break bad habit patterns and replace them with new healthy habit patterns. Even though all of life is change, we resist change with surprising regularity and unexpected intensity. Seek to make fundamental changes. Any changes you attempt will not endure until and unless they conform to your core beliefs. Real change is always a profoundly inside job. You can make the change; you can change virtually any and everything about yourself by taking one small step at a time.

The "Habits Change Process" takes you through a number of steps. The starting point is to evaluate yourself; it's to determine where you are by means of looking at what you do. In other words uncovering the habit patterns driving your life; in this case your nutrition.

Begin this nutrition change process in one of two places, whichever suits you best.

The first option is to approach this intellectually, deliberately and methodically. You may have kept a food journal a number of times. Do it again. This time however,

CHAPTER 6 NUTRITION: ONE STEP AT A TIME

as you catalog everything you put into your body over the course of a week (a full seven days) attempt to uncover how much of what you eat, or specifically what you eat, is habitual. In this case your food log or food journal becomes your habits log.

You might organize your food journal this way:

<u>Day of the Week</u>

Time	Food / Drink	Quantity	Craving	Circumstances

Time: might be time of day (7am, 9:15am, 12:20pm and so on) or by meal time (breakfast, morning snack, lunch and so on)

Food/Drink: this is whatever you consume or put into your body, solid or liquid.

Quantity: could be serving size (as in 8 ounces) or number of items (3 cookies) or if you are a calorie counter at heart

125

CHAPTER 6 NUTRITION: ONE STEP AT A TIME

you could list the amount of calories. Don't get bogged down on this detail.

Craving: record what you feel; the feeling which moved you to eat or drink whatever you consumed. Look for the trigger here. Did you consume something because of a hunger pang in your body? Or because of an emotional cue? Were you responding to a specific schedule (lunch break, etc.)? Or were you eating or drinking socially? The challenge with isolating a craving is sifting the body's signals for nutrients from emotional and social cues.

Circumstances: this is a notes field to ultimately record similarities in consumption patterns which upon closer examination will prove to be habits. List here some of those circumstances (struggling with a work problem, physically alone, etc.), contributing factors (other than the feeling, the craving) you identify as initiating consumption.

Your real task with the food journal is to be a detective. Don't be concerned so much with what you ate as with uncovering habit patterns. You will make progress; you will fundamentally change direction by changing habits.

After a full week of keeping track of what you consume extract from your log your "Nutrition Habits Inventory". These are your consumption habits. Then begin the work of changing those habits. Follow the "Habits Change Process" as you move forward.

I said you could start this process one of two ways. The first is by sorting out where you are. The second is to jump in by immediately changing one of those habit patterns undermining your health. In other words, if you've been to this rodeo before and you know you have a soda habit or that you are addicted to sugar, being immediately to STOP THE MADNESS.

CHAPTER 6 NUTRITION: ONE STEP AT A TIME

Instead of working through a formal habits inventory process focus on changing the one habit you know is setting you back. Work on one habit at a time until you have changed it, that is replaced that bad habit with a habit which serves you, a habit which properly nurtures your body.

The "Habits Change Process" still applies here. Isolate the habit you intend to change. Sketch out the habits cycle. Identify the trigger, the situation initiating the craving. Examine the actual physical process you execute automatically. And identify the reward, the satisfaction you get by flowing through that habit pattern.

The challenge with health and fitness is that nothing happens in isolation. Be aware your body adjusted to whatever habit patters, good or bad, you have established. Your body is attempting, to the greatest degree possible, to maintain an equilibrium; a status quo. The body is doing the best it can with the nutrients and toxins you provide. The body initiates cravings automatically in circumstances it senses as potentially sustaining equilibrium.

To change, counteract what your body has settled into. You created these conditions with the choices you made over the course of your lifetime. Your body has settled into workable routines, even unhealthy, ultimately detrimental routines, but the best your body could do given the circumstances. Acting to change these patterns is going to throw your body out of balance. Be ready for this hurdle.

The next concern changing nutrition and play habits is that while we feel "in the moment" what we feel is the result of what happens over time. How we feel in any instant is a product of both current circumstances and what has come before. Regarding nutrition, that craving you experience at 10:30 am may be more a result of skipping breakfast or

CHAPTER 6 NUTRITION: ONE STEP AT A TIME

consuming a donut at 7 am than it is the result of an overall energy deficit in your body. Your body, given your habits, has determined to maintain a certain blood sugar level. When you slip below that blood sugar level your body initiates a craving which it knows can be met conveniently by a soda. You have set a trap for yourself. Stop falling into the trap.

Changing nutrition habits is an "all in" undertaking. What you eat or drink now is going to affect how you feel later. While you work on individual habits recognize that what you do or fail to do now is going to have an impact later. Educate and prepare yourself for the challenges lying ahead. A comprehensive strategy will better prepare you to deal with the difficulties and obstacles you are sure to encounter on this road to a new healthy and vibrant you.

Determine to change the physical routine part of the habit pattern. Set yourself up for success.

First dig through your cupboards and your refrigerator and any food caches you have at school or work. Read all the labels. Get rid of anything containing trans-fats, high fructose corn syrup, or artificial sweeteners. Get rid of all highly-processed, high-calorie, high-sugar content items. Get rid of the cookies and the cakes, the chips and the soda, the ice cream and the candy. Clean out all the junk food. Now, before you go engaging once again in the battle of wills, just as important, perhaps more important than ridding your cupboards and frig of all of those processed toxins, stock up on viable replacements.

Prepare to Deal with Cravings

Have naturally flavored water readily available. Have nuts and berries, fruits and vegetables, low-sugar yogurts and natural jerky close at hand. The biggest challenge changing

CHAPTER 6 NUTRITION: ONE STEP AT A TIME

eating habits and dealing with cravings is planning and preparation. Have tasty, fresh, whole, natural substitutes ready and close at hand. Be smart, be prepared. Plan and prepare your meals and snacks ahead of time to ensure your success.

Eating healthy, just like engaging in joyful invigorating play every day, initially requires thought and preparation time. Make planning and preparation a habit too.

Making a lifestyle change requires thought and time. You must change your shopping habits, your food preparation habits, even your dining-out habits. Once you change those habits however, once you move from a highly processed diet that is slowly killing you to a fresh healthy diet you will see that being lean, fit and healthy is the better option. Being lean, fit and healthy is how you are meant to be. Make the change.

As you start down a new path, realize those cravings are going to come; no doubt about it. You must act. You still are going to be driven to satisfy an urge, to achieve a reward. Choose wisely. You don't always have to consume something; you could do something instead. If you do consume something, consume something to properly fuel your body. Have a healthy substitute readily at hand.

Changing nutrition habits is a holistic process. Work one habit at a time and set yourself up for success. Repetition is the name of the game. Ensure healthy alternatives are conveniently available. Don't expect perfection. You can eat sweets now and again. What you will find is that if you set yourself up for success; if you establish new conditions, adopt and nurture new habits; your body will change and you won't crave soda and sugar and toxins anymore.

CHAPTER 6 NUTRITION: ONE STEP AT A TIME

Your task is to guide and support. Your automatic pilot will take care of the details. Set the conditions and change to premium fuel.

Change your nutrition habits one step at a time. Out with the bad, in with the good.

Habit by habit, step by step a new, healthy invigorated you will emerge.

CHAPTER 6 GET OUT AND PLAY

Overcoming Resistance

We are accelerating toward the end of our program, the end of our time together. The entire point of this program is to expose you to high performance health and fitness habits. Why? So you can adopt high performance mindset, nutrition and play habits to turn your life in a new direction. When you employ high performance health and fitness habits your body automatically and naturally optimizes your health, your fitness and your performance.

With the right habits you can't help but become stronger, faster and fit.

In this section we focus once again on our theme of resistance and deliberately overcoming resistance during daily play sessions. We have stressed proper breathing; we have discussed warming up appropriately and working through a full range of motion. We have emphasized the simplicity of exercising with tools already at hand; your own body and gravity. We have explored incorporating simple tools, like kettlebells and balls, to spice up play sessions and add another dimension of challenge. And we have extolled the benefits of yoga and Pilates.

Our bodies are meant to overcome obstacles, hurdles: resistance. Our bodies are the vehicles which allow us to explore and experience this reality. The natural environment presents resistance from the very beginning. We must overcome resistance to move, to explore, and to grow. Overcoming resistance is part and parcel of life. The magic thing about our bodies is they will adapt; they will transform themselves to address and overcome the resistance they

CHAPTER 6 GET OUT & PLAY: OVERCOMING RESISTANCE

routinely face automatically, when given the right circumstances and support.

Take on the Challenge

A common strategy we human beings employ is to take the path of least resistance, the easiest route. Taking the easy route however, shortchanges our bodies. Our bodies are willing and able, are in fact eager to respond to the challenges of resistance. If we don't expose our bodies deliberately and intentionally to resistance, especially in this modern age of conveniences, if we don't systematically condition our bodies, our bodies will settle for the lowest common denominator. We will never achieve our full potential.

If you don't test yourself, if you don't push yourself you will never be strong, you will never build endurance and flexibility, you will never be as fit or as healthy as you could be. You must expose your body to resistance now in order to strengthen it. Properly prepared and properly conditioned, your body will serve you well. With proper conditioning your body can do extraordinary things. Condition it.

If you refuse to expose your body to resistance; if you refuse to challenge your body and overcome the resistance it needs to become strong and fit you will pay a price later. Choices, poor health and fitness habits, limit ability and mobility. By making bad choices you experience pain and fatigue in greater measure and you experience these discomforts sooner than you would otherwise. And, with poor health and fitness habits, you are more likely to put on excess weight and deal with all the problems carrying around additional pounds presents.

Your health and fitness habits are critical. And you don't need lots of money and gadgets and gizmos to play

CHAPTER 6 GET OUT & PLAY: OVERCOMING RESISTANCE

effectively. You just need an engaging spirit and the willingness to move every day.

It is possible to quite adequately exercise your entire body using just body-weight; no tools required. If you do have the opportunity, and most everyone has the opportunity, we have access to any number of tools to put our muscles and systems under the strain of resistance in focused and controlled ways. Using the proper tools we can build a body into a magnificent vehicle; one which will perform for many decades to come.

Here are some common and effective tools you can use every day to help build muscular strength and endurance.

Free Weights

Free weights come in a variety of forms; from dumbbells to barbells, from kettle bells to medicine balls; anything that has weight acts as resistance. Here again gravity comes into play.

Free weights may be used to isolate select muscle groups and systematically put them under tension; pushing or pulling, extending or contracting. Weights, like dumbbells, may be used to move through specific limited or full ranges of motion through single planes. Or weights may be used to challenge a wide range of muscles, again through limited or full ranges of motion, as in total body exercises through multiple planes (twisting, turning, bending and so on).

Weights are a useful tool to include in your playtime repertoire.

CHAPTER 6 GET OUT & PLAY: OVERCOMING RESISTANCE

Resistance Machines

Gyms and fitness centers offer a seemingly endless variety of machines designed to isolate single muscles or select muscle groups. You may be familiar with Nautilus and Universal brands, these machines have been around for decades. Most full-spectrum fitness facilities have one or more brands of resistance machines to help people strengthen muscles and improve endurance.

You don't need a fancy gym however, to optimize performance. Just put your muscles and your systems under resistance. The keys to effective resistance training are:

1) Breathing properly

2) Proper form and technique

3) Increasing Intensity (working the muscles enough to cause them to grow)

4) Adequate recovery

If you exercise correctly, for the appropriate duration and intensity, and given the proper nutrition, your body will respond automatically.

You have virtually an endless variety of tools to use to put your muscles through their paces and to the test. You can even use items you have around your house and yard to add to your kitbag of active play paraphernalia. You don't have to buy a thing. Use what you have. Make the most of what you've got.

Resistance Bands, Cords and Straps

Weights are bulky and heavy and resistance machines are, for the most part stationary. So here is one less-bulky tool to consider using to thoroughly exercise your body.

CHAPTER 6 GET OUT & PLAY: OVERCOMING RESISTANCE

Resistance straps, cords, or bands come in a variety of styles. Some are bands with handles, some are built into more complex machines and some are simply stretchy pieces of rubber or some synthetic fibers. These straps or bands have certain advantages over machines and traditional weights.

First, and obviously, cords, straps or bands are less bulky and are not difficult to store or carry around, say for instance if you travel. Straps or bands may be used in a variety of exercises and applications allowing you to put virtually every muscle individually or every muscle group collectively under tension, through a wide range of motion. And straps or bands, unlike free weights, are not only dependent on gravity. You can put your muscles under tension at various angles and through various ranges of motion. Free weights, in contrast, offer resistance in one direction: down.

A flexible band maintains tension throughout its full range of motion; both while elongating and while returning to its equilibrium or static condition. Controlled, deliberate movements through a wide range of motion using resistance straps or bands may prove to be a more effective means of putting your muscles under tension without the expense and bulk of buying a full set of weights, barbells, dumbbells, or resistance machines and all the accoutrements.

Bands and straps come in a wide range of resistance levels. With simple, creative adjustments you can increase or relieve tension to optimize the resistance you feel.

When using any exercise tool always execute proper technique. You can train your body, strengthen your muscles, improve your endurance and optimize your body's operating systems by using what you've got. Bands, cords and straps are inexpensive, effective resistance training tools.

Don't Resist Resistance Training

Resistance training, especially training which puts major muscle groups or your entire body to the test, has an advantage over every other type of physical activity. Overcoming resistance through a whole-body exercise taxes your muscles, your skeletal system, your cardio vascular system and all your other physiological systems uniquely in a way like no other movement does. A high-intensity, full-body movement triggers the release of a medley of health enhancing hormones you just aren't going to get any other way.

Every form of play, every form of exercise is a means of overcoming resistance. If you ratchet up the intensity and involve virtually all your physiological systems you significantly reduce the time it takes to play for optimum fitness. High intensity does not necessarily mean high-impact, high-speed or high-stress types of movements. Unless you want to be an elite athlete you can get all the benefits of whole-body, high-intensity exercise in one play session per week. One high intensity session per week allows you to devote all your other play sessions to releasing stress, moving and grooving, stretching and breathing; the things you must do to stay sane and happy and well.

It can be done. Your play program does not require more time. Thirty minutes of play a day provides untold benefits.

But for optimum results; to bring the pieces of mindset, nutrition and play together; to optimally engage all of your body's systems, execute a whole-body, high intensity resistance program once a week. Work up to incorporating

CHAPTER 6 GET OUT & PLAY: OVERCOMING RESISTANCE

this form of play into one session a week by first playing every day, by experimenting and testing systems, and over time by gaining exposure to a variety of resistance training programs. Work your way carefully up to high intensity.

Variety is the spice of life. I bet you haven't heard that before. Use programs that spark your interest and keep you wanting to play more. Resistance training is a lifetime activity. Overcome resistance on your terms now to make your body stronger. All your body systems will work better. And you will be able to overcome what life throws at you.

There are no shortcuts here. You will find more effective resistance programs and less effective resistance programs. Find a resistance program you can, will, and enjoy doing. And for maximum benefit and optimum performance, incorporate one whole-body, high-intensity resistance routine into your weekly play sessions.

You need not devote more than thirty minutes a day to play. Consistency, doing something every day, and intensity, taxing your entire body, are more important than duration. I would never however, discourage investing more time in play. Have fun!

Select something you can and will do routinely; then do it.

Don't resist this idea.

Develop the habit of overcoming resistance. I guarantee you'll be better for it.

CHAPTER 7 MINDSET

You Are Not Alone

If it is true: We're here to help others. What exactly then are the others here for?

Shouldn't they be here for us; to help us?

If all those people sharing our lives don't seem to be helping, if all those people we encounter on the highways and byways, in the hustle and bustle of life seem more of a hindrance than a help, maybe it's time to consider we're just not seeing the big picture, we aren't grasping the entire truth. Maybe they aren't the problem. Maybe our perspective is the problem. It takes great maturity and learning to understand that all things, events, encounters and circumstances are helpful. That includes accepting and embracing all those people.

As the population expands opportunities multiply. More people, more chances to connect, to give, to grow, to learn, to create, and to love.

We are not alone. We are not traveling alone. Life is a collective journey. We rely on other people, we need other people. And those other people rely on us, they need us.

Each individual has strengths and weaknesses, special gifts and talents. We are stronger, more intelligent, and more capable together than we can possibly be alone. We encourage each other, we inspire each other, and we support each other.

Life is Relationships

We are social beings. We cannot be happy unless we are connected and unless we are secure in those connections.

CHAPTER 7 MINDSET: YOU ARE NOT ALONE

We cannot be healthy without the help and cooperation of others. Our health and wellbeing, our fitness and vitality are encouraged by, supported by, and made possible by the people who surround us. Life is all about relationships.

High performance habits are those few key habits that give us the most leverage in life; the habits allowing us to perform up to our potential. Connecting with other people, genuinely, joyfully, is a lever habit. Connecting with other people promotes health and wellbeing. Connect with the right people, for the right reasons, and in the right way.

As social beings we are meant to be operating in a setting where we are connected, safe and secure, confident and capable, excited and optimistic. We are meant to be performing at an extremely high level, but upon encountering the weight and resistance of the environment we often lose our way. We fumble around in the dark. We allow fear to dominate. Fear begins to get the upper hand and we settle. We determine just getting by is good enough. Anything else isn't worth the effort; isn't worth the risk. Other people are here to encourage us not to succumb.

Examining the lives of the greatest achievers in history we discover all the opportunities they enjoyed, all the opportunities for achievement and success came by way of other people; no exceptions. Inspiration comes from spirit, from the *Source*, from *God*, more often than not though, it is delivered and served up by way of other people. As we are guided by, encouraged by, inspired by and supported by forces outside of what we could possibly define as our physical bodies we are guided by, encouraged by, inspired by and supported by other people.

How we manage relationships matter. Our interpersonal skills matter. Our social habits matter. These

CHAPTER 7 MINDSET: YOU ARE NOT ALONE

matter a great deal. The quality of the company we keep and the quality of the connections we make directly impact health and fitness.

In this jungle of time and space it's easy to fall victim to fear. It's easy to begin to believe we're lost, separate and alone. If we don't believe we have skills and talent and power we scurry around looking for a safe place to hide. We hope for a quick and merciful end to the troublesome journey. If on the other hand, we sense we have some power, some skills, and some talent to potentially compete and perhaps gain an upper hand, to take what we want, we will. But our talent, our skill, even our power, only goes so far. In the end power, skill and talent always fall short. We secure our success and happiness by cooperating and collaborating with other people.

Connect and Engage

This entire *High Performance Health and Fitness Habits* program emphasizes to be happy, to be healthy and fit, nurture habits of feeling, thinking and acting which engage your automatic pilot. We engage our automatic pilots in one of two primary ways. The first is by way of personal intrinsic motivation; our attitude and mindset. When we've got attitude and mindset right we are connected and driven; not driven to compete and dominate, but rather driven to explore and experience, to express more life, to fulfill our potential. With the right attitude and mindset we are focused and capable of traveling fast.

The second way to engage our automatic pilot also happens to be the most common means of impeding our own progress. This is a way we potentially set ourselves back. We engage our auto-pilot through the influence of the people around us; our social support network. We are influenced,

CHAPTER 7 MINDSET: YOU ARE NOT ALONE

for better or for worse, for richer, for poorer, by the people in our lives, from the very beginning.

The people who have surrounded us, and who surround us now, have influenced who we have become. They have influenced our core beliefs; the beliefs determining what manifests in our lives.

Take stock of where you are now.

Are you surrounded by confident, positive people, people who see opportunity, are willing to grow, and are going somewhere?

Do you have a network of positive, supportive people around you to help you advance, grow and become?

Healthy people, fit people, balanced and centered people deliberately associate with and surround themselves with positive, uplifting, capable people. Healthy and fit people focus on building, nurturing, sustaining and maintaining loving supportive relationships.

You Get What You Give

A word of caution here. Before we start down the path of judging people and ending relationships consider this thought. What we see in other people is often a reflection of ourselves. The criticism we level with the most emotion, with the most conviction, is usually a veiled attempt to excuse ourselves. We see, expressed through someone else, the very same weakness we possess. Often to relieve ourselves of responsibility, and in a misguided attempt to mete out punishment, we judge and attack others.

So remember, all people, all circumstances, all events are helpful, and change is an inside job. To change the world out there, we must change our selves. Everyone you

CHAPTER 7 MINDSET: YOU ARE NOT ALONE

associate with serves a purpose; a positive purpose. What you perceive as getting from those people you hold in a negative light is not their true nature. What you get just may be a reflection of you; your attitude and your approach to them.

How do you routinely present yourself to people you consider negative? The problem may not necessarily be them. If we are honest with ourselves the problem may be us.

Do you have a positive, life-enhancing support network?

If you don't have a supportive, inspiring network, it's time to establish a network-building, a relationship-building habit.

To be healthy and fit, to be successful and happy; to have more, do more and become more surround yourself with and routinely associate with, positive, growth minded, and uplifting people.

Positive, growth minded people will help you keep a positive attitude and stay in a growth mindset. Positive, growth minded people will help you and encourage you to take care of your body with proper nutrition, rest and relaxation. And positive, growth minded people will provide you opportunities to take risks, get out of your comfort zone, try new things, and play joyfully.

The right support network of people will push you, will challenge you, and will test you. Respond to the challenge. Get out of your comfort zone, starting meeting new people, begin building and nurturing your growth network. You will not regret that choice.

CHAPTER 7 MINDSET: YOU ARE NOT ALONE

Quality Matters

Success, succeeding, health and fitness are not about the number of people you have on your team. Advancing in the right direction is about the quality of the people you have on your team and the bonds of trust and respect you form.

Altering the course of relationships may prove to be the most difficult habit to change in this entire health and fitness habits journey. But nothing, no change of habits you make is going to prove to be more rewarding.

This means potentially changing how you support and interact with even the people closest to you. This means expanding your network. You owe it to your family and friends; your closest confidants and supporters; to evolve the nature of your current relationships. Take responsibility for this change.

If you believe a relationship is on balance negative, that is has a negative influence on you, than your task is to change yourself and bring something more positive to the relationship. With children this change effort is one hundred percent your responsibility. With other adults, reforming a negative relationship takes work and ultimately cooperation from all involved. Building new relationships and salvaging and reshaping long-standing relationships are noble and rewarding undertakings. Get to it.

You may end up having to distance yourself from some people, people who just aren't ready or willing to embrace a new course. Every individual makes his or her own way. It's not ours to judge. Distancing ourselves from negative people, doesn't mean shutting them out. Family is family; blood or otherwise. The task dealing with negative relationships is to bring positive energy to bear. In time, even after a genuinely concerted effort, some people are

CHAPTER 7 MINDSET: YOU ARE NOT ALONE

unwilling or unable to absorb positive energy. If this is the case in a relationship you are intending to reform, keep channeling positive energy. Negative people will tend to avoid you. Always encourage others to grow. This habit will serve you well.

The energy of others influences health and fitness. Associate and surround yourself with positive, growth minded people. Begin by changing your habit of mind. Exhibit a positive attitude and a growth mindset. Once you have a positive attitude and growth mindset you will naturally gravitate toward like-minded people and start reforming and refreshing your network. Then take the process one step further. Make the act of connecting with and interacting with positive, growth minded people a habit. You will be better for it.

Succeeding, which includes health and fitness, is not a solo affair. Health and fitness depend on a number of factors which you manage. Relationships can serve or set you back. To ensure your health and fitness build loving, mutually supportive, life-enhancing relationships.

CHAPTER 7 NUTRITION

Take Aim

What are you aiming at?

What are you hoping to achieve with *High Performance Health and Fitness Habits*?

Are you worried about your weight?

Are you obsessed with ever increasing clothing sizes?

Are you embarrassed by the way you think you look?

Does moving cause you aches and pains?

Does climbing a flight of stairs make your heart race?

What we are after with *High Performance Health and Fitness Habits* is not defined by weight or size or appearance. *F*ocus on what matters: how you feel. If you feel good, if you are healthy and fit, weight, size and appearance are just a detail, a detail taken care of for you automatically.

How you feel is your gage for life. How you feel is an indicator for whether or not you are headed in the right direction; going where you want to go, experiencing what you want to experience and accomplishing what you want to accomplish. How you feel tells you whether you are taking care of body and whether or not you are training and maintaining properly.

If you generally feel good, energetic and vitally alive you are on the right track. If you generally feel bad, are tired, stiff or sore or if you avoid doing things because engaging in any physical activity is a chore, you are on the wrong track.

CHAPTER 7 NUTRITION: TAKE AIM

It comes down not to how you look, what size you are or how much you weigh. What matters is how you feel.

We didn't begin this program setting goals. We haven't even mentioned weighing and measuring and testing ourselves to determine how much weight to drop or how much strength, endurance or cardiovascular fitness to gain. You wouldn't explore a program like *High Performance Health and Fitness Habits*, and you most assuredly wouldn't get this far in the program, unless you are dissatisfied with the condition of your body or you are searching for some answers. Here is that drum beat again:

We are what we repeatedly do.

Excellence then, is not an act, but a habit.

By nature we human beings are "goal setters". We define and establish goals automatically. The vast majority of goals we set are proximate, that is they are short-term, situation dependent, and usually driven by a physical desire or craving. We all are goal setting and goal achieving machines. We feel hungry; we grab some food. We feel tired; we sit down. Though you might not usually equate these actions as formal goals they are goals we set and work towards consistently. Some goals we set are conscious, most are unconscious.

Goal Achieving Machines

The good news is we are goal achievers by nature. The bad news is we often don't set the right goals. We are all achievers; some of us however, don't achieve much of any good. We get in our own way because of what we determine to do. We usually, mostly, typically define short-term, feel-good goals. We don't aim very high, because we don't need

CHAPTER 7 NUTRITION: TAKE AIM

very much and aspiring to greater achievement demands more energy, more commitment and more effort.

Regarding nutrition habits what are the right goals?

Eliminate any harmful or hurtful inputs. Adopt nutrition habits providing your body with the optimum fuel; what it needs to stay healthy.

Health is a matter of sustaining all systems in proper working order. All parts and systems of the body are healthy when each is doing what it is supposed to do optimally, and the systems are working together in concert, collaboratively. When all component parts are contributing to the adventure we are operating at or near our potential.

When we are healthy we have the most options. We feel good. We feel vibrantly alive. We are ready to advance.

The primary way to measure your health and fitness is to listen to your body.

How do you feel?

Do you feel good; energized, strong, and capable?

Do you have aches and pains?

Are you suffering discomfort and distress?

How do you feel when you put your body to the test?

Can you move through multiple planes of motion?

Can you handle and overcome increasing loads of resistance?

Can you physically move far and move fast?

If you can't move without straining yourself something is wrong. You are not as healthy and fit as you can be.

CHAPTER 7 NUTRITION: TAKE AIM

Long-term health and fitness rests on the foundation of core beliefs. Core beliefs influence the goals we set, the choices we make, and the habits we develop. If you make the right choices, have the right mindset, fuel your body properly and play vigorously, consistently, your built-in automatic pilot we keep you flying high and straight and far.

Health and fitness are simple enough. Do the right things consistently, repeatedly until those actions become habits; things you do automatically, without thinking.

What Is the Right Direction?

How do you know if you are heading in the right direction?

How will you know when you have arrived?

Do you want to do more than the minimum?

Do you aspire to greatness?

The first and most important gage is how you feel. But listening to your body may not be enough.

If you prefer to see results and measure progress imagine this chance process as adopting a whole new high performance habits lifestyle.

Start with a self-assessment. Evaluate your current state of health and your overall condition. Determine where you are and then use this record to see just how far you travel as you change your habits.

Some of these assessments you can make on your own. Some are best measured with the help of a partner, and some may require the aid of medical or diagnostic professionals. Be as complete and comprehensive as you want to be.

Check, test and record these data points:

CHAPTER 7 NUTRITION: TAKE AIM

Height

Weight

Body Composition (determine body-fat percentage and water weight)

Determine your ideal weight (Don't sweat this. Everyone is different and the ratio of muscle to fat affects body weight. The more muscle you have relative to fat, the more you will weigh and this is a good thing. So treat this ideal weight figure as purely a theoretical gage.) A number of systems or formulas will provide you an ideal weight and each system or formula offers a different calculation and will arrive at a different result. The Hamwi equation is one simple, well known method for calculating ideal weight: Females: allocate 100 pounds (lbs.) for the first five feet of height, then add five pounds for each inch of height over five feet. As an example, a woman who is five feet, five inches tall (5'5") would have an ideal weight of 125 lbs. Males: allocate 106 pounds (lbs.) for the first five feet of height, then add six pounds for each inch of height over five feet. As an example, a man who is five feet, ten inches tall (5'10") would have an ideal weight of 166 lbs.

Resting Heart Rate

Blood Pressure

Determine your Basal Metabolic Rate (BMR) (This is for those calorie counters. BMR is the number of calories your body burns at rest to perform all your normal systemic functions. Your BMR accounts for approximately 60% - 75% of your calorie needs. BMR depends on: overall health, size and relative muscle mass, and age.) (Don't sweat this one unless you really enjoy the numbers.) The Mifflin St.

CHAPTER 7 NUTRITION: TAKE AIM

Jeor Equation, listed here, is considered the standard when it comes to calculating BMR, but a number of other equations exist. Handy calculators are available online.

Men

BMR = (10 x weight in kilograms) + (6.25 x height in centimeters) – (5 x age in years) + 5

Women

BMR = (10 x weight in kilograms) + (6.25 x height in centimeters) – (5 x age in years) – 161

Measurements: waste, hips, thighs, biceps, calves, forearms, chest

Record current clothing sizes (pants, shirts, dresses, skirts, suit jacket)

Conduct a biochemical assessment (blood and urine tests) to record such things as fasting glucose levels, cholesterol levels, iron status, vitamin D status, and sugar, ketones, and urine specific gravity.

List any food allergies or conduct a food sensitivity / food allergy assessment.

List any genetic conditions, chronic diseases or physical limitations (arthritis, diabetes, etc.).

List all medications and supplements you currently take.

Conduct a fitness test to measure cardiovascular fitness, muscular strength, muscular endurance and flexibility. (Some of these tests are simple with few movements (push-ups in a given time (say one minute), sit-ups or crunches in a given time, run a given distance timed (say one mile), and stretch (as in the stretch and reach). Some fitness tests

CHAPTER 7 NUTRITION: TAKE AIM

however, can be quite involved and comprehensive. Do your research and settle on fitness measures best conforming to your fitness goals.)

Conduct a physical skills test to measure agility, balance, coordination, power, and reaction speed. (Like with the fitness test, some skills tests are simple and straight forward others are more comprehensive and involved. Again do your research and settle on physical skill measures best conforming to your physical skill goals.)

Regardless of how detailed and or comprehensive your self-assessment is, if you want to measure progress this list is your starting point. Your end state or goal is health and fitness. Goals only work when you do. Set goals and take action.

Health is a state of being; of feeling good and feeling energized. Your entire body and all its systems, are working at their best, as they should.

Fitness is a measure of being able to subject yourself to the rigors of moving through this reality and overcoming resistance. The more fit you are the more resistance you can overcome for longer durations and with greater skill.

Improving health and fitness are most dependent not on setting goals but on taking consistent action. Whatever goal or goals you establish, whether to weigh a certain amount, to fit into a certain size of clothing, to be able to run a given distance in a certain time or to lift a certain weight, ensure they move you to act. Effective goals are a means to develop good habits.

Thinking, strategizing, planning and preparing all happen up front. Take aim. Set your goals. Visualize

CHAPTER 7 NUTRITION: TAKE AIM

yourself the way you intend to be. See yourself as a new healthy you. Think, imagine, and visualize what you need to do to make yourself take action. Leverage your desires and the cravings your body generates to get going.

Eat healthy. Substitute fresh, whole, natural foods for those highly processed, high-sugar foods and drinks. And play consistently. Make your body work for you, for your best long-term self-interest; for optimum health and wellbeing; not against you.

Becoming healthy and fit and having a great body is more a factor of what happens in the kitchen and dining room than what happens in the gym. Remember the analogy we used early on. You would never put sand in the gas tank of a performance automobile or airplane and expect that vehicle to perform. The same holds true for your body.

Get your mindset right. Make smart choices and act appropriately. The act appropriately part of the health and fitness equation is to develop healthy eating habits and to play vigorously every day.

The target you are aiming for could not be clearer.

Take aim and then fire; your goal is nothing less than a new you.

CHAPTER 7 GET OUT AND PLAY

Getting Up to Speed

If you have been involved in the exercise side of the health and fitness industry you have seen a variety of formal exercise systems come and go. We discussed those machines, gadgets and gizmos before. New-fangled ideas, methods, gadgets and gizmos serve practical purposes. Of course every new idea is a potential source of profits, but more than that, each idea offers variety and an enticement for acting.

Not every new idea, gadget and gizmo is a fad. The fundamentals: mindset, nutrition, and play, are the fundamentals, but all those methods have a place. Whether jumping rope, dancing, standing on mechanical surfboards, riding mechanical bulls, dangling from suspension systems, or climbing walls and conquering obstacles, every system offers benefits. The biggest benefit is inspiring action. Evaluate new ideas, gadgets and gizmos by these criteria:

1. Does it entice you to move?

2. Does the gadget, gizmo or system offer resistance in a way to improve strength, endurance, and flexibility?

3. How much does it cost and will it last (at least as long as my interest)?

Exercise Duration

For optimum health and fitness you do not have to spend hours playing. Playing thirty minutes a day vastly improves health and fitness. Current health and fitness research points us to our roots. The natural lifestyle of most human beings for thousands of years was long periods of rest

CHAPTER 7 GET OUT & PLAY: GETTING UP TO SPEED

(hours) and long periods of moderate activity (again hours) interspersed with short bursts of intense whole-body activity.

By playing thirty minutes a day you will be more fit than average. If however, you want to optimize your fitness; that is maintain a high level of muscular strength and endurance, have increased cardiovascular capacity, and be able to perform through a full range of motion with superior flexibility; you must work smarter than most for those thirty minutes.

World class athletes, men and women who win the races, carry the loads and capture championships, are deliberately, intelligently and specifically training five or more hours per day. To be the best at something you must devote time, energy and talent to that something in a determined, consistent way. But health and fitness, high performance health and fitness, not world class athlete level of performance, are something you are designed for. Health and fitness come naturally when you exert yourself properly.

Intensity is the critical component of the fitness formula, not time. Most people are bombarded by competing demands. We devote time, energy, and talent to everything from recreation and entertainment, to childrearing and home maintenance, to earning a living and leisure pursuits. We have a nearly endless variety of activities from which to choose. To excel we must manage intelligently.

If you want big results for little time; those thirty minutes of play a day; up the intensity at least once per week. To devote less time to play increase the intensity.

You may have questioned a lack of focus on traditional cardio in this program. Typical cardio conditioning is running, biking, swimming or using an elliptical machine. Cardio is an activity engaging large muscle groups, like legs

CHAPTER 7 GET OUT & PLAY: GETTING UP TO SPEED

and buttocks, and taxing the cardiovascular system. For most people cardio is a matter of sustaining a set pace for a predetermined duration.

Endurance athletes spend hour upon hour engaged in their sport of choice. Their bodies adapt over time to the meet the demands placed upon them. A body attempts to maximize efficiency. If you however, are out of shape and intent on getting your body back to its natural state of being lean, fit and healthy, long bouts of cardio are not the way to go. A more natural and effective cardiovascular form of play is to move the entire body under the added resistance of weight. Whole-body, high-intensity play offers the best results for the time committed.

Whole-body, high-intensity, low-impact exercises are the play activities of choice. These are the Bentley of fitness activities and you only need to push yourself to the limit once per week. Your body needs plenty of recovery time after a whole-body, high-intensity workout. If you move from low impact to high impact speed adds another dimension. Also with speed comes a greater potential for injury.

Unless you intend to be an athlete don't focus on speed. Only once you are confident in your flexibility and range of motion should you venture into high impact or speed workouts. Moving too far, too fast is a recipe potentially for disaster. In the interest of exploring the full spectrum of options however, let's increase the intensity.

Power Equals Force Times Velocity

To minimize the time you devote to active play work harder. To increase the resistance you subject your body to, and to incorporate more muscle fibers, exert more force by moving at a high velocity. As with all forms of overcoming

CHAPTER 7 GET OUT & PLAY: GETTING UP TO SPEED

resistance, and assuming proper technique, your body will automatically adapt to increasing loads. Moving fast and working hard you become stronger and endurance improves.

To be an endurance athlete, long bouts of cardio are necessary, but intensity matters here too. To lose weight and tone up, consider other types of exercise; more whole-body, higher intensity exercises. You will see greater results for a short time allotted to play.

An advantage of high-intensity, whole-body play is it leverages the body's natural systems. If your hormones are out of whack, the fuel you provide is critical to getting your systems functioning properly again, but even beyond that is your type of activity. Engaging in whole-body, high-intensity play; activity using your core, your chest, shoulders, arms and neck and your buttocks and legs; taxes your cardiovascular system, muscle strength and endurance, skeletal and other systems in a more complete way than running or walking.

An activity working multiple systems more intensely is the more beneficial type of play. Lower intensity activities rarely meet the physiological threshold to trigger an optimum hormonal response. Whole-body, high-intensity play triggers the flow of repair, rejuvenation and growth hormones to improve health and fitness.

If you have been watching the exercise landscape you have probably seen high-impact, high-intensity programs proliferating. Some people really enjoy high-impact, high-intensity play: games, sports, exercise programs and recreational pursuits. High-intensity, high-impact is certainly an option. Just proceed with caution.

CHAPTER 7 GET OUT & PLAY: GETTING UP TO SPEED

Plyometrics

Plyometrics is also known as jump training. The key with plyometrics is making muscles exert maximum force in the shortest interval of time. The goal with plyometrics is to increase both speed and power. Training focuses on extending and contracting muscles in an explosive manner. The primary resistance is usually provided by body weight however, weight may be added through a variety of means: free weights, bands, weight belts and so on. Imagination is the only limit.

Plyometrics are an intense way of training. You jump; jump up, jump forward, back, and side to side using one or both legs. Plyometric movements may be done from the floor, in other words using explosive extension and contraction techniques like in a push up or through a burpee or squat thrust. Again you are only limited by your imagination.

Plyometrics incorporates most if not all of the body through explosive movements. Executing the movements in rapid succession taxes the cardiovascular, musculature, skeletal and other systems.

Conditioning yourself to take on plyometrics is a long-term goal. Don't start your play program here. If your goal is to be really, really fit, incorporating plyometrics into your play regimen will accelerate your progress.

Combat Training

If you have been watching, you likely have noticed a variety of combat type training programs rise in popularity recently. These programs range from traditional martial arts to hybrid exercise varieties. Traditional martial arts incorporate a total person focus; mind, body, spirit; into the

CHAPTER 7 GET OUT & PLAY: GETTING UP TO SPEED

training regimen and system of discipline. The discipline of martial arts is a habits formation process. Martial arts training helps practitioners master the habits of mind and body for optimum health and fitness.

Traditional martial arts range from low-impact, low-intensity to high-impact, high intensity varieties. Look for a martial arts style to match your style; one which is in line with your goals. As with yoga and Pilates look around. Try some things. Test some things. Keep on playing.

The combat type training used for fitness classes are systems typically employing martial arts moves. These systems offer a whole-body workout. Participants use arms and legs, hands and feet and rely significantly on their core for balance, speed and power.

Basic moves include kicks: front kick, side kick, back kick, crescent kick, hook kick, axe kick and so on. Strikes range from straight punches to jabs to hooks to uppercuts to knife hand and ridge hand strikes and back-fists and hammer-fists, elbow and knee strikes. Combat training includes defensive techniques like blocks and throws and grappling and so on. Some of these programs, traditional and hybrid, incorporate tools; weapons; for added skill development. A full routine of combat type training executed at high intensity works the entire body from head to toe.

Many gyms or home training systems, using DVD's or streamed recordings, incorporate up-tempo, invigorating music into their combat routines. The music adds to the intensity and the fun. A high intensity combat type workout more than covers the bases for taxing your systems. They are worth a try.

CHAPTER 7 GET OUT & PLAY: GETTING UP TO SPEED

A traditional martial arts discipline is a complete mind-body training system; much like yoga. You can choose between high and low impact varieties. A typical hybrid combat training program tends to favor high-impact movements but is usually performed in an engaging way. Look around. The programs are fun and might just be the right system to take you to the next level of personal growth and development. Try it, you might like it.

High Intensity Interval Training (HIIT)

The last potential play activity to leave you with is the current rage of high intensity interval training (HIIT).

Ratchet up your play session intensity over time; over months. As you shed excess pounds, and as your health and fitness habits change, your body will make this happen automatically. As you begin to see yourself as someone who is fit or getting fit and who is capable, continue pushing yourself.

High intensity interval training is an exercise sessions to engage your entire body and all your physiological systems in an intense way for a relatively short period of time, say ten to twenty minutes. Warm-up and cool-down are additional time. High intensity interval training aficionados have demonstrated that just one or at most a couple of HIIT sessions per week is all anyone needs to work their muscles, tax their cardiovascular system and trigger a positive hormonal response. One or two HIIT sessions per week maintains total body fitness.

A typical HIIT session consists of a series of fast-moving intervals (could be as few as three or as many as ten or more). An interval lasts a predetermined time, say three to five minutes. Participants rest between intervals for a predetermined time, say from thirty seconds to two minutes.

CHAPTER 7 GET OUT & PLAY: GETTING UP TO SPEED

An interval consists of one or more different moves (calisthenic type moves: burpees or squat thrust, push-up, jumping jacks, pull-ups, and so on) each done for a prescribed number of seconds. The combinations of exercises and times are limitless. People are devising new routines and new combinations of exercises every day. Many are body-weight only, and many incorporate all the aids, gadgets and gizmos we have talked about in this program and more. The point with HIIT is to push yourself, tax your muscles and cardiovascular system and to trigger a favorable hormonal release. Just be careful not to injure yourself.

Ease In

Work up to incorporating one whole-body, high-intensity, low-impact session into your play routines per week. But, and I can't emphasize this enough, above all else, don't overly concern yourself with the specific type of activity you are engaging in when you play. The point of play is to release stress and joyfully engage your body. If your mindset habits are right and your nutrition habits are right, actively playing every day is enough. You will move in the right direction.

Traditional cardio, that grinding mile after mile on the treadmill or the road, is not necessarily your ticket to optimum fitness. As a matter of fact, bouts of cardio, long duration steady state exercise may be counterproductive for weight loss and your overall health and fitness. If you are trying to maximize results for the time you commit to play you have other options.

Develop play habits to first and foremost. Ensure you execute; play every day. Aim to make one play session per week more intense by incorporating a whole-body, high-

CHAPTER 7 GET OUT & PLAY: GETTING UP TO SPEED

intensity activity. Done properly you will cause your body to overcome resistance and activate your endocrine system to promote recovery and growth.

You can, of course, incorporate high-impact, high-intensity, whole-body activities into your play program. Plyometrics is on the more intense end of the intensity scale. A traditional martial art or combat type workout engages your entire body and adds a whole other dimension to your play repertoire. Adding speed ups the intensity. HIIT is on the intense side of the scale.

Increasing resistance is the key to improving performance. Proceed intelligently. Listen to your body. Don't overdo it. Proper technique and appropriate rest and recuperation are essential.

As daily play becomes a habit your body will adjust to new demands and then plateau. Increase the resistance and increase the intensity to keep making progress. Minimize your time commitment by working your entire body in high intensity activity.

As you get stronger and faster, more capable and more fit, you will be able to do more than you thought. Keep exploring your limits. Keep pushing yourself. You may discover no end in sight. Recognizing a world of possibilities is a good place to be.

CHAPTER 8 MINDSET

You Know What to Do

Everything about life, the environment, the conditions, the support systems are stacked in our favor. We have entered into an extraordinary environment, a place to flourish. We have ready access to all the resources we need to survive and thrive. We have people around helping, supporting, inspiring and motivating us. We have a litany of forces beyond the physical world encouraging and guiding us. We are meant to succeed, to blossom and prosper. We have been given more than enough in a world with more than enough to do something truly extraordinary, something exciting, something creative and something uniquely our own.

You have not been cast off alone in the darkness. You have the capacity, the capability, the gifts and the talents to rise to extraordinary heights. Excellence is not for the select few. You can become anything. You have the power to set your course. Health and vitality, fitness and wellbeing are not beyond you. You are meant to be healthy and fit and vibrantly alive. Make the most of the opportunity. Go as far as you can as fast as you can. Make the right choices.

You have the tools to embrace the fullness of life. First and foremost is the power of thought. Thought is the link from the material world to the infinite beyond. Each body comes with an automatic pilot built-in. That automatic pilot, once properly engaged keeps us flying high and straight and far. And you have an energy conservation mechanism known as a habit process. Set yourself on the right path; leverage the power of habits to thoughtlessly and effortlessly keep moving forward.

CHAPTER 8 MINDSET: YOU KNOW WHAT TO DO

You are meant to live life to the fullest, to have life abundantly, and to fulfill your potential. You have the resources, the assets and the support to go places and do things. Let yourself go and get going.

Health and fitness, really all aspects of achievement and success, are a matter of adopting habits to ensure success. Habits carry us far and move us fast. Choose, develop and nurture the right habits to go where you want to go. The power is in your hands. Select and employ the assets available to you. Make the choices to set your course and then act.

You can choose to be a bystander. You can choose an easy path, a path of comfort ruled by fear. Or you can choose to fly high and go where others fear to tread.

Choose a path to test yourself and challenge yourself; a path which brings out your best. Leverage the tools you possess to become all you can be.

Make Health and Fitness a Habit

Everyone uses their energy conservation device: the habits process. Too few actually deliberately employ the habits process for high performance. Use the habits process to ensure your health and fitness, your wellbeing and vitality.

You recall, the habits process is comprised of four parts:

1) A stimulus, which generates

2) A craving, which initiates

3) An action routine, which intends to achieve

4) A reward.

STIMULUS > CRAVING > ACTION > REWARD

CHAPTER 8 MINDSET: YOU KNOW WHAT TO DO

By repeating the feeling-action-feeling sequence enough we eliminate the need to think to get the feeling we are after. We use habits to feel, automatically and thoughtlessly.

How we feel, how we think, and how we act are quite frequently habits. We set ourselves up to respond to certain triggers and get a pre-determined result. Change habits, change lives. Employ the right habits, the best habits and change course. New habits change what we do, what we believe and ultimately who we become. Put the power of the habits process to work. Engage the lever habits of mindset, nutrition and play.

Core Beliefs

You have more opportunities than you could ever take advantage of during a single lifetime. You have access to more resources than you could ever employ. You have more gifts and talents, skills and abilities then you could ever fully realize and exploit. And you are more loved and supported than you could ever even imagine. Why then are you stuck?

We launch our life journey with such confidence and enthusiasm. Somewhere along the way however, we start forming a worldview. This worldview becomes our foundation for life. Our worldview, our core beliefs, orient us for superstardom or flaming failure. This choice of words is intentionally overdramatic. In life you are guaranteed to succeed. You cannot fail. You have the power to choose your own course and make your own way. Is your foundation solid or is your life built on rubble?

Establishing core beliefs is a matter of experience and interpretation. Life is a feeling-action process. We feel. We judge. Many of us prefer ultimately to protect ourselves from pain and sorrow. We begin to believe the world is a

CHAPTER 8 MINDSET: YOU KNOW WHAT TO DO

threatening, dangerous place and that we are alone, disconnected, incapable and unsure. And we begin to believe we have no purpose being here. Clinging to these core beliefs we determine to take what we can and muddle through. We relinquish the promise and potential of a grand and glorious life. We choose to believe a lie and then we allow that lie to carry us to dark and desolate places. Staring into the abyss despair consumes the light. This is **not** how life is meant to be.

Believing we are in a welcoming world, a safe and forgiving environment; that we are connected and capable and strong; and that we have a reason for being sets us on a very different course.

Core beliefs matter. They are the foundation we build our lives upon. If your core beliefs are not allowing you to achieve your potential you must change them.

Core beliefs, having been built over a life time, are very powerful. But there is always hope. You have the power. Change your core beliefs by changing what you do. Change your habits to produce new results. New results will create a new reality. Seeing new results will change your perspective. Changing your perspective will influence core beliefs and your progress will accelerate.

Lever Habits

A lever habit is a habit process providing disproportionate leverage. Lever habits influence broad swaths of experience. MNOP are lever habits. The primary lever habit to develop is a mindset habit. Develop a positive attitude and growth-oriented mindset. Attitude determines altitude. Life presents you with all you need, with more than enough; open yourself to the blessings you enjoy. Embrace the adventure.

CHAPTER 8 MINDSET: YOU KNOW WHAT TO DO

Use the habits change process to change your mindset. Enlist the help of trusted allies and reliable friends. Your power of thought, though not absolute, is the premiere power you control. Making the best choices is a function of your mind: your mindset. Focus on developing a positive attitude and growth mindset. This one habit will set you up for success.

Habits Change Process

The mechanics of the habits change process are pretty straight forward:

Know where you want to go and in which direction to head.

Determine which habits are setting you back.

Make a plan to break bad habits and develop good habits.

Get to work.

The biggest challenge in any change process is maintaining the motivation to change. We human beings as a rule hate change. We cling to what we know tenaciously. You need a reason "why", a reason to change, bigger than all the resistance you can muster. Focus first on motivation. Determine why it is you want to change. Hold that vision of "why" before you as you engage in the habits change process and keep moving forward.

Tackle one habit at a time.

Sketch out the habit sequence for the bad habit you intend to change.

Determine the trigger, the craving, the action routine and the reward (that feeling you seek).

CHAPTER 8 MINDSET: YOU KNOW WHAT TO DO

Then work out a new action routine.

Keep the trigger and the reward exactly the same; change what you do.

Practice your new habit routine until you are comfortable with how it feels.

Write down a comprehensive habits change plan.

Set a time and date to begin your new habit routine and fix a duration; how long you intend to focus on building your new habit.

Figure out how you are going to get back on the horse when you fall off; when you settle back into your old habit routine.

Recruit some support. Bring some people you trust into the process. Ask them not to judge but to support you through the change.

Then execute.

One by one, habit by habit make small changes. Reinforce success. As you succeed changing small habits turn your attention to developing a lever habit. Once you empower a lever habit things will change significantly. Get your mind right. Change your eating habits. Play; invigorating, joyful play; every day. Each of these lever habits is mutually reinforcing. They go together; they reinforce each other.

MNOP habits will put you on the fast track to health and fitness. This will, in turn, accelerate your progress to success and happiness. You are guaranteed to succeed.

CHAPTER 8 MINDSET: YOU KNOW WHAT TO DO

Manage Stress

Life is filled with stress, with resistance. To make your way, overcome stress and resistance. Be careful though, too much stress can be overwhelming.

We face external stressors in the environment, microscopic biological stressors and social stressors. But the most dangerous stressors of them all are the stressors we generate within our minds. We set goals, we determine timelines, we aspire to be admired and love. We set expectations. When life does not match our expectations we generate our own anxiety. We generate our own stress.

We can't avoid all stressors. Eliminate stress where you can and leverage stress where you must. Don't tie your own hands. Don't fix your expectations about other people or about circumstance. Don't cling tightly to specific outcomes. Life is bigger than that. God has a bigger plan. Trust in that plan.

Mitigate and manage stress. Learn to recognize and deal with environmental, biological, social and psychological stressors. Take time to think and pray and meditate. Play; joyful, invigorating play is quite possibly the best stress relief known to mankind. Develop habits of feeling, thinking and acting to manage stress. Use stress as a motive for action not an excuse for inaction. The less we cling the less stress we endure. Let yourself go, and then keep on going.

A Collective Journey

A journey of a thousand miles begins with a single step. If you want to go fast go alone, if you want to go far go together.

Life is a long and rewarding journey. You have a far way to go. The rewards along the way are beyond your

CHAPTER 8 MINDSET: YOU KNOW WHAT TO DO

wildest expectations. Your travel agent – God – has set the conditions for your optimum benefit, your optimum comfort and your optimum achievement. You never travel alone.

Embrace the collective of life. The most rewarding, the most profoundly moving aspect of this experience is love. Love is the mutual embrace of all beings, of all creatures, of all that is.

You are here to travel, to explore and experience. You are here to learn and to grow. You are here to create and contribute. You do all of these; explore and experience, learn and grow, create and contribute; in communion with other people.

Build and maintain your love network. Nurture and support other people. Embrace the collective journey.

You, we, all of us will go far by traveling together.

With the right habits you can go as far as you are capable of going. Think. Put your mind to good use. Choose and choose wisely. And act joyfully.

There are no limits to what you can have, do and become.

CHAPTER 8 NUTRITION

Eat Fresh

There is an old adage you are likely familiar with: "Knowledge is power." This is a valid maxim, but upon closer examination we realize the statement is incomplete. Knowledge represents potential power. Knowledge is only power if and when it is applied, and applied properly.

Knowledge itself, the assembling, organizing and storage of information is primarily a passive undertaking. Often, most notably in a formal education setting, acquiring knowledge takes place in our heads. Acquiring knowledge is passive in the sense that we, for the most part, absorb and sort information. We attempt to make sense of it, we might even go so far as to understand, but for the most part, we let it wash over or pass through us. We accumulate and organize information. Look at your bookshelf or on your technology (smart-phone, tablet or computer), at databases and archives, at notes and message logs. We have been exposed to and work with huge amounts of data, reams and reams of information. What have we done with it all?

We covet knowledge. We eagerly pursue it. We stack it up. We want knowledge because we believe knowledge is power. Knowledge is not power until we do something with it.

Life is a feeling–action adventure. Life is what happens, not to us, but through us. To participate in life means to take action: to do something. There is no getting around it. We must do something with what we know.

Knowledge can open doors. Knowledge can expand horizons. Knowledge can be the key, the gateway to every

CHAPTER 8 NUTRITION: EAT FRESH

good thing and blessing. But we must apply knowledge appropriately to realize any blessings. We must act.

Think of our formal education system. Think of all the facts and figures, the ideas and concepts you have been exposed to since kindergarten and elementary school. If you went on to college or post-graduate education you have considered, manipulated, and likely accumulated quite a storehouse of knowledge. Have you applied all that knowledge?

Most people have smart-phones these days. If knowledge is power, the advent of the smart-phone has made the individual extraordinarily powerful. Through a smart-phone we have access to information, the likes of which most of us could not even have imagined just a generation ago. Think of the power at your fingertips. With all this power in the hands of individuals we should be advancing at lightning speed. Are we? Do you think most people feel more powerful, more capable, better off?

We have the power in our hands. We have the potential of immense knowledge. We just aren't using that power very well, if at all.

Knowledge is power only if we use it, if we apply it.

Do We Know? Do We Care?

Advancing in life requires action. Life is action. To move in a given direction we must "do something." We must act. How we act, what we do, the choice we act on, makes all the difference. To close the loop on this knowledge metaphor: the way we act, the specific knowledge we apply is what produces a result. It is what moves us through life.

CHAPTER 8 NUTRITION: EAT FRESH

Life, living, is a verb, but not just any verb it's a specific verb we choose. Applying knowledge generates power, generates motion. We make life happen when we apply what we know.

I hope you are with me, because we are going to make a leap here. And you may be wondering, "What the heck does this have to do with nutrition and nutrition habits?" Please bear with me.

Motivation and knowledge are connected. Let me illustrate.

Progress, movement in a given direction, and ultimately success, requires two elements: motivation which drives action and a course or direction to take. Knowledge lays out our options for what course or direction to take. Knowledge informs our choice.

We might classify people relative to motivation and knowledge as operating from one of four stations. For "motivation" I'll use the word "care" or "caring". For "knowledge" I'll simply use the word "know".

We could apply these dimensions of being across virtually all areas of life in general but they are particularly useful when it comes to considering health and wellbeing.

Pick a specific category, a specific area of interest. People either "care" or they "don't care". Caring here means something that will move them to act a specific way. People either care or they don't care about virtually any and everything. Then, people either "know" or they "don't know;" that is they either possess, have access to or understand something, or they don't.

CHAPTER 8 NUTRITION: EAT FRESH

Some people who care also know and some people who care don't know. Some people who don't care know and some people who don't care also don't know.

This same model applies to health and fitness; to habits of health and fitness. Some people care and some people don't. Some people know and some people don't.

Which one are you?

The answer to these questions:

Why am I not healthy and fit?

How do I become healthy and fit?

are pretty simple and straight-forward. We are not fit and healthy because we are not making the right choices. We are not fit and healthy because we are not employing the right habits. We are not fit and healthy because we are not fueling our bodies with fresh, whole, natural foods. We are not fit and healthy because we are not playing; moving our bodies, engaging in joyful, invigorating play every day.

And how do we become healthy? By making the right choices. By guiding and supporting our bodies to properly activate our automatic pilots. By fueling our bodies with fresh, whole, natural foods. And by engaging in joyful, invigorating play every day.

Life Is Stacked in Your Favor

You have everything you need to be fit and healthy, vibrant and vitally alive. You have access to the knowledge you need. Apply it.

The key to fueling our bodies, the key to achieving, sustaining and maintaining health and fitness is providing our bodies the right nutrients, in the right quantities, at the

CHAPTER 8 NUTRITION: EAT FRESH

right times. This is not something to lose sleep over. Choose, develop and nurture the right eating habits.

Nutrition does not have to be confusing. The guidelines to follow are very simple. Just apply the right knowledge to leverage your habits process. By adopting the right eating habits nutrition, health and wellbeing will be as good as they can be automatically.

The worst of all mistakes is not that we don't know: it is "knowing" something that just isn't so. Beware misinformation. Beware of those well-funded interests appealing to your emotions and base motivations (pleasure and convenience); the ones claiming to offer healthy alternatives. Beware of what even government sources recommend. Government agencies operate with any number of agenda's. Truth is often sacrificed for other expediencies.

Fresh, whole, natural foods; not processed or man-made; are the essential fuels for your body. Change your nutrition, your eating habits. Develop the habit of reaching for real foods when you need them. Break your sugar addiction if you have one. Stop rationalizing that only calories matter and dismiss the notion that fat is the enemy. Diet sodas, diet anything, if diet really means artificial sweeteners and man-made fats, are never the answer.

Eat fresh. Stop the madness of sodas and processed foods. Eat a plant-based diet consisting primarily of non-starchy vegetables. Consume natural proteins (not proteins stuffed with antibiotics and genetically modified grains) and include natural fat as a staple of your diet.

Rely on the right information. Educate yourself then go a step farther. Take action. Apply the knowledge. When you do, when you apply the right knowledge in the right

CHAPTER 8 NUTRITION: EAT FRESH

way, when you finally adopt healthy habits you will be on the right road. You will begin to realize your true potential.

You are meant to be happy and healthy and fit. You can go far and travel fast. You can experience everything you want to experience. The way is simple. Choose the simple path, the best path, the fresh path.

We hurt ourselves when we either don't know or don't care. Now you know.

Start down a new path.

CHAPTER 8 GET OUT AND PLAY

Play Some More

We have covered a lot of ground in *High Performance Health and Fitness Habits*. We have drilled on those MNOP habits: to be healthy and fit, to live up to your potential, adopt right mindset habits. Develop habits fueling our bodies with the best nutrients possible. And make a habit of staying active, of getting out and playing. With health and fitness it really is a matter of use it or lose it.

When we employ the right habits we engage our autopilot appropriately. Our bodies automatically adjust to ensure our health, to manage our weight, and to adapt to overcome resistance.

To be trim and toned, strong and fast, agile and flexible play every day. Use your muscles; engage all those physiological systems. Nobody can do this for you. This is and has to be your task, your mission, your goal. Get out and play every day. You will be healthier happier for it.

Variety Is the Spice of Life

Activities to engage in range across a broad spectrum from the traditional, what we might call labor or work, to what is typically referred to as exercise, to unconstrained play. What you do impacts your body: your muscles and your systems. More important than what you do however, is that you do something. Life is not a spectator sport; you are a player, engage.

Make daily play a habit. Make getting out and playing such an ingrained part of your daily routine you just won't feel right unless and until you have released all your cares and worries and moved your body. Elevate your heart rate.

CHAPTER 8 GET OUT & PLAY: PLAY SOME MORE

Engage in some friendly competition. Or enjoy roughhousing with some young ones.

We hear a lot about taking ten thousand steps a day, with gadgets and gizmos monitoring every move. Those gadgets and gizmos have their place, but just remember the key to health and fitness is not to chain yourself to a gadget rather it is to free yourself from bad habits and empower yourself with the right habits.

Through this *High Performance Health and Fitness Habits* program we have emphasized various types of activities you might incorporate into your play routines. Think about your goals and desires and your preferences. There is no, one-size-fits-all here. As a matter of fact, the activities you enjoy are probably going to evolve and change over time. That's okay; that's terrific; that's as it should be. Just don't ever stop. You are either moving forward, overcoming obstacles, adapting and growing, or you are withering away. Life is too precious and time is too short to squander.

You have a body capable of fantastic things. Develop habits; ways of living; encouraging, allowing really, your body to perform at its best. Given the right conditions, the right inputs and the right support your body will take care of the details and take care of you.

We introduced the elements of fitness early: body composition, muscular endurance, muscular strength, cardiovascular endurance, and flexibility. Active play helps improve each of these elements. Active play helps improve agility, balance, coordination, power and reaction speed as well.

Each individual has a different level of natural ability. But everyone can improve their fitness and their physical

CHAPTER 8 GET OUT & PLAY: PLAY SOME MORE

skills. Practice doesn't make perfect; practice makes us better. The way to ensure we are always moving forward is to make the practice of building, maintaining, and sustaining our health and fitness a habit.

Over the course of these eight modules, or chapters, or sections, or sessions we have specifically worked through typical types of exercise programs. Your daily play session can be just that, play. It can be running around playing tag or hide and seek. It can be engaging in an organized activity like a sport. Tennis anyone? Or basketball? Or soccer? Or racquetball? Or volleyball or any host of active, engaging games. Get your entire body involved. Move through a broad range of motion. Tax your cardiovascular system; get your blood flowing, your heart pumping; pull in some fresh air.

The activities you engage in could be group or solitary pursuits: things like walking or hiking, running or biking, swimming or rowing. If you are not as fit as you want to be now, begin instilling this daily play habit as a social routine. Get other people engaged; you might rotate among different groups and different activities on different days. You are much more likely, first, to engage in an activity if you have a social commitment and, second, to push yourself, at least a little bit, when you are with other people. Keep the social factor in mind as you develop and reinforce your play habits.

At the beginning of every play session warm up your muscles and loosen your joints. Get your blood flowing as you gradually raise your body temperature. Deliberately and at times methodically stretch out your muscles, loosen them up. We can always improve flexibility, but we have to work, or rather, play at it.

CHAPTER 8 GET OUT & PLAY: PLAY SOME MORE

Your core, all the muscles of your back, chest, abdomen, buttocks and so forth are critical to maintaining your body posture and ultimately your overall condition and health. Move your body constantly through its full range of motion. You use your core constantly; focus on activities to strengthen it. Explore the possibility of using kettlebells or medicine balls or other devices, gadgets and gizmos to expand your full-body play repertoire.

Don't become enamored by gizmos and gadgets however. We don't have any legitimate excuses not to play. You have everything you need; a body and the resistance of gravity; to achieve optimum health and fitness. Two-thirds of American adults have more than enough of what they need to provide resistance for muscles and bones, joints and ligaments and all their bodily systems. Don't think you need a fancy gym and an expensive gym membership to get fit. Do the best you can with what you've got.

For maximum results do the right exercises, the right activities; overcome resistance in the right way, using proper technique, at the right intervals. Listen to your body, but don't give in. Push yourself. If you combine the right activities with proper nutrition and a positive growth-oriented mindset, you literally can't help but get better. Your body will automatically and quite naturally become fit.

Yoga and Pilates are a great addition to any play program. These are two types of activities, systems really, which facilitate the mind-body connection. Both yoga and Pilates deliberately work the entire body in a way to relax and free the mind. If you haven't tried these, yoga and Pilates, go out and find a studio or look for free classes in your area. You won't regret it.

CHAPTER 8 GET OUT & PLAY: PLAY SOME MORE

Breathe as You Overcome Resistance

The play component of fitness has two recurring themes. The first is learning to breathe. We are one with the environment; we need fresh air in our bodies. The more effectively we breathe, bring in fresh air to energize and revitalize our systems, the healthier and happier we are. The second recurring theme is overcoming resistance. We covered body-weight exercises and resistance training.

We human begins are designed to overcome resistance. Resistance is the nature of reality, of our environment. Our bodies naturally adapt to effectively address the resistance we routinely face. Play with greater intensity; not every day, but at appropriate intervals; say once per week. Put your body to the test. Feed it what it needs and ask it to perform; your body will respond. I guarantee it.

This entire process of becoming fit and healthy is not time consuming, or it doesn't have to be time consuming unless you want it to be. It's not expensive, or it doesn't have to be unless you want it to be. Being fit and healthy is a choice. It is a choice you make based on the habits you develop, adopt and nurture. If you develop the right habits; mindset, nutrition and play habits; you will automatically, without thinking about it, without stressing about it, you will automatically develop and maintain a high performance body. Then you can do what you want to do. You can go where you want to go. You can have more, do more and become more.

Develop high performance health and fitness habits; MNOP habits; and fulfill your potential.

You have nowhere to go but forward.

We are waiting to watch you soar.

Afterword

We are creatures of habit. Habits have brought us this far and habits have made us who we are. Are you flying as high, as fast and as far and you want to be? How well is your automatic pilot managing your flight?

As I stated at the very beginning, *High Performance Health and Fitness Habits* is not so much a motivation program, a nutrition program or an exercise program as it is a habits change program. You control your life only when you control what you repeatedly do.

We are what we repeatedly do.

Excellence then, is not an act, but a habit.

You have everything you need to be healthy and fit. You are meant to be healthy and fit. You can have more, do more and be more. All you need is enough desire to act. You know what to do. Change your habits to make health and fitness automatic. Engage your health and fitness auto-pilot. You don't have to worry about every little detail. The details will all be taken care of for you. You just have to pick a direction and get moving. Listen to your body. Work with your body. Guide and support and challenge your body and it will respond. Focus your mind, feed your body, and move with joyful abandon.

Your health and fitness are your responsibility. No one can do this for you. Take advantage of human nature. Don't be a victim. Take control. You are master of your fate; you are captain of your soul. Put your energy conservation device, your habits process to good use. Develop and nurture a positive attitude and growth mindset. Fuel your body with premium fuel. And get out and play every day.

Once you make health and fitness a habit, once you make moving forward a habit, you will soar. You are guaranteed to succeed!

Words are a poor substitute for communicating what is best expressed through the example of action. You are left now to go out and test this habits change process in the real world; in the laboratory, the playground that is life. If you apply the principles, if you make incremental changes, you will succeed. Experiment with an open mind and your perspective will broaden, your attitude will change and your faith will deepen. With enough faith you can move mountains. Great things are in store for you. Believe!

Scott F. Paradis

Appendix A
Health and Fitness Defined

HEALTH (Y):

- State of being free from illness or injury; the condition of being sound in body, mind, or spirit; the general condition of the body (Merriam-Webster Dictionary); State of complete physical, mental and social well-being and not merely the absence of disease or infirmity (World Health Organization); Condition of optimal well-being (The Free Dictionary)
- State or condition of optimum performance; all systems are functioning properly; person is capable, confident and sure, energetic and vitally alive (HPH&F Habits)

FITNESS:

- Quality or state of being fit; capacity of an organism to survive and reproduce (Merriam-Webster Dictionary); Quality of being suitable to fulfill a particular role or task; degree of adaptation to an environment (Collins English Dictionary)
- Measure of conditioning relative to maximum potential or capacity; elements of physical fitness: body composition, cardiovascular endurance, muscular strength, muscular endurance, and flexibility (HPH&F Habits)

AUTOMATIC PILOT:
　　The body's innate control system regulating and integrating the functioning of physiological systems; acts to ensure survival; attempts to maintain optimum physiological balance given inputs and conditions; adapts to overcome resistance; conforms to environmental conditions; responds to stressors (HPH&F Habits)

CORE BELIEFS:
　　Personal beliefs about: the state of the world (dangerous or safe), one's abilities (connected and capable or disconnected and incapable), and one's place in the world (purpose for being); orientation to life profoundly influencing choices which in turn drives habit formation (HPH&F Habits)

ENERGY CONSERVATION DEVICE:
　　Innate HABITS FORMATION PROCESS minimizing an individual's expenditure of energy by alleviating the need to think when satisfying an urge (HPH&F Habits)

Appendix B
High Performance Habits Change Process

We human beings are creatures of habit. We rely on habits to simplify our lives. Habits either help us fulfill our potential or hinder our progress. To become all we have the potential to be we must choose, develop and nurture the right habits.

Making a change requires three elements: motivation, a new focus, and a willingness to act. Habits however, are routines we build and reinforce over time. Each individual habit is governed by a cue or trigger and a coveted reward, a feeling. To deliberately change habits employ a deliberate change process.

DELIBERATE HABITS CHANGE PROCESS

1. Assess Current Habits: evaluate each habit to determine if it hurts or helps.

2. Prioritize Habits to Change: determine where to start.

3. Identify Habit Cycle Elements: sketch out habit cycle (cue, trigger > craving > action routine > reward/feeling) for those habits that must change.

4. Select New Habits to Adopt: develop a new vision.

5. Make a Plan: include the "big picture" and implementation details.

6. Test: run through the new habit routine a few times; adjust plan.

7. Enlist Support: get help from people you can count on and trust.

8. Execute: implement the plan, change a habit; adjust plan; keep going.

Step 1: Assess your current habits

- Complete a **Habits Inventory**.
- Evaluate each of your habits (+ positive, - negative, / neutral) to determine which habits must change.
- Highlight those habits you intend to eliminate or replace.

Step 2: Prioritize the habits to change.

- Review you **Habits Inventory**.
- Create a prioritized list of habits to eliminate.

Step 3: Produce a Habit Cycle sketch for the habit you intend to change.

- Sketch, actually draw out, the **Habit Cycle** for the habit.
- Identify the "Cue" / "Trigger" (the stimulus initiating a habit cycle).
- Identify the "Craving" / "Desire" (a feeling).
- Describe the "Routine" (the state or mood (for a feeling habit cycle) or the thought pattern (for a thinking habit cycle) or the action sequence (for an action habit cycle) that is the heart of the habit process).

- Identify the "Reward" (that something, which ultimately is a feeling).

Carefully conduct this detective work. The routine part of the habit cycle is the easiest part to identify. The Cue, the Craving, and the Reward are not necessarily easy to determine. Take some time to identify the true motive. Do not assume you're eating because you're hungry. The real reason may be that you are lonely or tired or upset or facing a challenging obstacle. Dig into each component of the habit cycle and discuss details with someone you trust to help sort it out.

Step 4: Select a new action routine to replace the bad habit.

- Select new habits to adopt. Specify the new action routine, the new habit.
- Test the new routine. How does it feel? Does the new routine generate a positive outcome? Describe the outcome in detail.
- Write out a vision statement for this new habit. What will life be like once you adopt the new habit routine? What are you intending to achieve? Focus on and stress "WHY", what is motivating about this change.
- Build toward adopting high performance lever habits.

Step 5: Develop the specific change plan.

- You've identified the habit to change and sketched out the Habit Cycle for that habit. You've selected a new routine, tested it, and envisioned a new you after adopting the routine. You have a clear goal and vision statement written out.
- Select a new habit implementation start date (when you are going to start).
- Specify the length of time you will focus on adopting the new habit routine. This could range from one week to 90 days.
- Think through and write down what you are going to do when you relapse; that is when you fall into your old habit routine. This is a means of starting again, not abandoning the effort.
- Determine who specifically you are going to enlist to help you through this change process.

Step 6: Run another test. Get familiar with the new habit routine. Believe you can change.

Step 7: Enlist support. Get your family members, friends and coworkers on board.

Step 8: Execute. Implement the plan.

Once you succeed with one habit move on to the next one and keep going. It's like climbing a ladder one rung at a time.

Step by step, habit by habit, create a new you; a new life.

ABBREVIATED HABITS CHANGE PROCESS

1) Choose a bad habit to replace.

2) Dissect the habit cycle of that bad habit. Specifically identify the circumstances that trigger a craving; specify the craving; define the action routine you execute; and identify the reward you receive. The REWARD IS ALWAYS A FEELING. Dissecting and identifying the components of a habit cycle is not as straightforward as it may seem. The craving and the reward may not be driven by what you might expect.

Think of a hunger pang example. Stress or emotional angst is often a trigger for craving sweets. The feeling of hunger may have nothing to do with a depletion of energy stores within your body. And as for the reward: a cupcake will provide some energy in the form of a sugar high, but that reward, the calories from the sugar, may only serve as a substitute for the satisfaction (THE FEELING) you get from both the taste of the sweetness and that temporary energy surge from the sugar. Or sometimes you may be looking to make a social connection by snacking with someone (ANOTHER FEELING). Neither the craving nor the reward in this case has anything to do with fueling or sustaining the systems of your body. Be watchful for emotional cravings and rewards. These are the ones to steer you wrong most of the time.

It is easier to move through this habits change process if you don't try to change everything all at once. Keep some things constant. Trying to change everything about a habit will not work. You could try to avoid triggering circumstances. You could try to achieve new rewards. But these are not really eliminating the bad habit. Focus on changing the routine; the action sequence you thoughtlessly have come to execute as the foundation of that habit. Life is a feeling–action process, change the action.

3) Determine a new action sequence to engage when feeling that craving and seeking that feeling reward. Practice the new action sequence. Then practice the sequence again and again.

4) Think through the details. Work through a deliberate planning process to change the bad habit. A written plan is not as important as carefully and deliberately thinking through the process. Resolve to recognize the trigger and the craving initiating that bad habit. Think through how friends can help. Set a specific start date and time to begin, and commit to executing the new habit process for a given number of days: 30, 60 or 90 days. And think through how you are going to reset when you fall back into the old habit pattern. Run another test. Execute the habit action sequence again and again. Really feel how the process is going to feel.

5) Enlist some support. Get some people you trust and rely on to help you execute and stick to your new habit routine.

6) Execute. On the appointed date and time initiate the new habits process. Stick with it. Over time you will develop a new habit.

Once you have eliminated one bad habit start the process again for the next habit to eliminate. Build toward adopting a level habit and your progress will accelerate. You will be actually changing core beliefs, in turn changing multiple habits.

Appendix C

Recommended Reading

If you are like me it takes some time and some repeated exposure to ideas for the truth to finally sink in and result in action. You can find thousands of books on the subjects of health and fitness, and millions of data points in books and articles, in databases and research reports, on and off line. If you care to look, you can find information to corroborate everything presented in *High Performance Health and Fitness Habits*. The key to your success however, is actually taking action. If you need more details as you begin to act, as you begin to change your habits, especially relating to nutrition, I refer you to three outstanding sources. Each of these authors will point you to an even broader array of references.

The Self Health Revolution by J. Michael Zenn

The Calorie Myth by Jonathan Bailor

Primal Body, Primal Mind by Nora T. Gedgaudas

You do not need to learn everything; just the right things. Good luck!

Appendix D
Feedback Request and Contact Information

You have put in a lot of time, energy and effort working through this program. You have a unique perspective to offer. Please help me help others get healthy and fit. I need your feedback on the strengths and weakness of **High Performance Health and Fitness Habits**.

Please send me, Scott F. Paradis, an email with your thoughts.

Here are some questions to help formulate feedback. Please don't feel constrained by this list:

What did you like LEAST about **High Performance Health and Fitness Habits**?

Was the program worth your time? Yes or No. Why?

Which idea or ideas did you find most useful / helpful? Why?

Would you recommend this program to others? Yes or No. Why?

What can we include or improve to enhance the implementation or change process component of the **High Performance Health and Fitness Habits** program?

Email your feedback to Scott@c-achieve.com.

If you would like me to speak to your group about ***High Performance Health and Fitness Habits, High Performance Habits*** in general or another **Success 101 Workshop** offering or if I can help you in some way please send me an email or call and leave a voice mail at:

(703) 772-3521

Be sure to leave contact information and I'll get back to you as soon as possible.

Thank you!

About the Author

Scott F. Paradis is a student of life and a seeker of ultimate truth. Striving to simplify the complex he studies human performance and potential through the disciplines of economics, business, human relations, communications, politics, philosophy, religion, athletics, and health and fitness. He intends to discern simple, enduring truths: the wisdom of life. Only once something is made simple can we, do we, truly understand.

A native of New Hampshire, as of this writing Scott lives in northern Virginia where he concluded a 30-year career with the United States Army. He is married to a shining star, the former Lisa Newcombe, and has two extraordinary adult children: Merideth and Mitchell.

Attempting to lead by example Scott helps people live full and fulfilling lives. He helps people dream big and build faith by establishing life-affirming habits of thinking, feeling and acting. And he helps people relate to others and life in positive, fulfilling ways.

Scott retired from the Army at the rank of colonel. In addition to varied stateside assignments he completed tours in Europe and the Middle East. He served as a National Security Fellow with the John F. Kennedy School of Government at Harvard University and as a National Defense Congressional Fellow with the United States Senate. He holds a Master of Science in Administration from Central Michigan University and a Bachelor of Arts in Sociology from the University of New Hampshire.

Scott's personal aspiration is for his life to be a message of hope, an example of faith, and an expression of love as he works to do the best he can with what he's got.

Acknowledgements

Everything I have done, everything I do, and everything I am yet to accomplish is made possible by the loving and supportive people who surround me and by those that are drawn into my awareness. My success is made possible by God's inspiration and the genius and generosity of countless other people.

For Lisa, my wife, and my two terrific children, Merideth and Mitchell, and all my family and friends I am forever grateful. I am truly blessed having wonderful people in my life.

To past sages, modern day prophets, and those searching diligently to express truth through insightful words and faithful examples I extend my most heartfelt thanks. The courage, commitment and sacrifice of men and women who embrace the opportunity that is life inspire me. I pray that the words etched on these pages might inspire you to take on laudable challenges, endure worthwhile hardships, and fulfill what I know to be limitless potential.

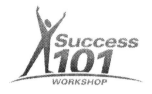

Success101Workshop.com

Success 101 Workshop is all about improving **performance** and helping people **live life to the fullest**. In our inspiring presentations and engaging workshops we focus on the fundamentals while striving to simplify the seemingly complex.

If you want to learn a task, if you want to improve, if you want to master something, focus on the fundamentals. Once you master the fundamentals there's no stopping you.

Through consultations, presentations and workshops, online courses and published insights ***Success 101 Workshop*** shows individuals how to live exhilarating lives of outstanding achievement and helps teams succeed beyond expectations.

We throw open the curtains obscuring simple truths. We help people see things the way they are and then imagine how great things could be. Then we set them on a new course.

Success, in business and in life, is not a matter of commanding irresistible power and employing overwhelming resources, it is a matter of doing the best you can with what you've got. You have more assets at your disposal than you know. By relying on your natural abilities and learning and leveraging the fundamental principles of success you can change your body, your mind, your business: your life. Yes you really can!

You have potential you haven't yet begun to tap. Contact us now, we can help.

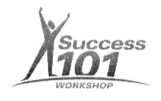

Available from:
Scott F. Paradis
Success101Workshop
Success101Workshop.com
&
Cornerstone Achievements

Books:

High Performance Habits Health and Fitness Habits
Engage Your Health & Fitness Auto-Pilot

High Performance Habits
Making Success a Habit

How to Succeed at Anything
In 3 Simple Steps

Success 101 How Life Works
Know the Rules, Play to Win

Promise and Potential
A Life of Wisdom, Courage, Strength and Will

Warriors Diplomats Heroes, Why America's Army Succeeds
Lessons for Business and Life

Look for these online courses offered by Scott F. Paradis:

High Performance Health and Fitness Habits, MNOP Habits

High Performance Habits, Making Success a Habit

Success 101 How to Succeed, Focus on Fundamentals

Money, The New Science of Making It

Success 101 How Life Works, Know the Rules, Play to Win

High Performance Leadership, Fundamental Leadership Habits

Loving 101, Making Love a Habit

Be, a Messenger of Hope, an Example of Faith and an Expression of Love

Contact us to schedule a customized presentation, a consultation or a performance oriented workshop:

High Performance Habits & High Performance Health and Fitness Habits

Success 101 How to Succeed, Focus on Fundamentals

High Performance Leadership, Fundamental Leadership Habits

Money, The New Science of Making It

Courtesy of 2015

Mount Vernon Athletic Club
7950 Audubon Ave
Alexandria, VA 22306
703-360-7300
iwant2bfit@mtvac.net
www.mtvac.net